DON'T KNOW MUCH ABOUT JOINTS

THE HIP

IRA KIRSCHENBAUM, MD

Images by The Medical Multimedia Group

DTC HEALTHCOM

Published by DTC Healthcom, LLC

405 Tarrytown Road, Suite 1390

White Plains, NY 10607

Text Copyright © Ira H. Kirschenbaum, MD, 2014

Images Copyright © Medical Multimedia Group 2014

ISBN-10: 1493720856

Printed in the United States of America

Without limiting the rights under copyright reserved above, no part of this publication may be reproduced, stored in, or introduced into a retrieval system, or transmitted, in any form or by any means (electronic, mechanical, photocopying, recording, or otherwise), without the prior written permission of both the copyright owner and the above publisher of this book.

The scanning, uploading, and distribution of this book via the Internet or via any other means without the permission of the copyright owner and the publisher is illegal and punishable by law. Please purchase only authorized electronic editions and do not participate in or encourage electronic piracy of copyrightable materials. Your support of the author's rights is appreciated.

Note to Readers

This book is intended for information purposes only. Hopefully it adds to your current knowledge about the subject matter and stimulates you to learn more. The diagnosis and treatment of all medical disorders is best left up to medical professionals.

TABLE OF CONTENTS

Introduction **14**
    What is this book about? 14
    How do I read this book? 14
    What if I have more questions? 14
    Why did you write this book? 15

General Questions About Joints **16**
    Why does someone have joint pain? 17
    what are some of the more common conditions that cause joint pain? 17
    What exactly is a joint in the body? 18
    Do all joints move? 18
    That doesn't make sense to me. How does a joint not move? 18
    Does it matter whether some joints move and some joints don't move? 18
    What types of joints are there in the body? 18
    What type of joint is a hip joint? 19
    What type of joint is the knee joint? 19
    What type of joint is the shoulder joint? 20
    What type of joint is the elbow joint? 20
    What type of joint is the wrist AND HAND jointS? 21
    What type of joint is the ankle joint? 21
    What types of joints are in the foot? 22
    What makes joints so smooth and cushiony? 23
    I have heard about joint lubrication. Is there really such a thing? 23
    Where does joint fluid come from? 23
    Why does cartilage lose its effectiveness? 23
    What does infection do to the cartilage and the joint? 24
    What does inflammation do to the cartilage and the joint? 24
    What does an injury do to the cartilage and the joint? 24
    What does aging do to the cartilage and the joint? 24
    What is arthritis? 25

How do I know a joint has arthritis?.. 25
What are the differences between an x-ray, MRI, and CT scan?... 25
Are there different degrees of cartilage loss or is it there one day and gone the next?.. 25
What does an x-ray show in arthritis?.. 26
What are some of the other ways to find out what type of joint problem I have?... 26
What are some of the general ways to treat joint problems?......... 27
When you say I can treat myself, what does that mean?................. 27
What are the common types of prescription medicines I take for arthritis"?.. 28
Do exercise and physical therapy work for arthritis?....................... 28
Does my weight have anything to do with arthritis or joint pain?
.... 28
What types of doctors treat which types of joint problems?......... 28

General Questions About The Hip 30
What and where is the hip joint?.. 31
Are there other things besides the cup and ball that are part of the hip joint?... 31
What is the labrum?.. 32
Are hip ligaments important?.. 32
What do the muscles around the hip joint do?.................................. 33
What are the tendons around the hip joint?....................................... 34
What is the hip bursa?... 34
If I were standing and looking at myself in the mirror and wanted to point to my hip joints, where would they be?................................ 34
What are the more common problems that cause pain in the hip joint?... 35
What is arthritis of the hip?... 35
What causes arthritis of the hip?.. 36
What type of hip problems in children can lead to hip arthritis as an adult?... 36
What is developmental dysplasia of the hip?..................................... 37
What is Legg-Calvé-Perthes Disease of the hip?................................ 37
What is Slipped Capital Femoral Epiphysis of the hip?.................... 38
At what age does hip arthritis affect people?..................................... 39

What does an x-ray of arthritis of the hip joint look like?............... 39
What is a fracture or a broken hip?... 40
What does an x-ray of a fracture or a broken HIP OF the hip joint look like?.. 40
What are other problems of the hip joint?.. 41
What is avascular necrosis? 41
What causes avascular necrosis? 42
What is hip bursitis?.. 42
What causes hip bursitis?.. 43
What is a labrum tear?.. 43
What is hip impingement or femoroacetabular impingement? ... 43
How important is it for me to actually know why I have hip pain? 44

Treatment of Specific Hip Problems 45
Hip Arthritis 46
What are some of the non-surgical treatments of hip arthritis?.. 46
Do any of these treatments reverse arthritis or build cartilage?. 46
How do I change my activity level to help my hip arthritis?......... 46
Does using a cane actually work? 46
What are anti-inflammatory medications?.. 47
What are Tumor Necrosis Factors (TNFs)?.. 47
What are steroids?... 47
Are anti-inflammatory steroids the same as the steroids we hear about that athletes take to improve performance?........................ 47
How are steroids given?... 47
What are some of the names of various anti-inflammatory steroids?... 47
What are the differences between all these brands of steroids? . 48
What are the positives about steroids by mouth?.......................... 48
What are the negatives about steroids by mouth?......................... 48
If there are so many negatives about oral steroids, then why even take them?.. 48
What are the positives about steroid injections into joints? 48
What are the negatives about steroid injections?........................... 49
What type of injections can I get for hip arthritis?.......................... 49
How does a cortisone injection work?.. 49

Is there a limit to the number of cortisone injections I can get? .. 49
What is a hyaluronic acid injection? 50
How do hyaluronic acid injections work for arthritis of the hip? 50
Does hyaluronic acid build cartilage? 50
Is there a limit to the number of hyaluronic acid injections I can get for arthritis of the hip? 50
What are NSAIDS? 51
How do NSAIDS actually work? 51
What is over-the-counter medication vs. prescription medication?
.... 51
Is there really a difference between over-the-counter anti-inflammatory medications and prescription anti-inflammatory medications? 51
What are NSAID creams or ointments? 52
What are some of the problems with NSAIDS? 52
Do all NSAIDS have the risk of upsetting the stomach? 52
Besides NSAIDS, what are the more common pain relievers for arthritis? 52
What are some of the problems with narcotic pain relievers? 52
What are some of the nutritional supplements that are being sold for arthritis? 53
Do glucosamine and chondroitin sulfate actually work? 53
If there are no scientific studies proving the value of these supplements, then what should I do? 53
Does physical therapy work for arthritis of the hip? 53
What kind of surgery exists for hip arthritis? 54
Labrum Tears **54**
Are labrum tears serious? 54
Are all labrum tears painful? 54
If a labrum tear is the cause of pain, what is the treatment? 54
What if rest does not work? 54
What type of surgery is there for a labrum tear? 55
Hip Impingement (Femoroacetabular Impingement) **55**
What is hip impingement or femoroacetabular impingement? 55
What exactly is the problem in FAI? 56
What is the treatment of FAI? 56

Why don't surgeons just do hip replacement as the first treatment for FAI? 57
Does FAI eventually go on to more severe hip arthritis that will NEED HIP replacement? 57
Avascular Necrosis **58**
How is avascular necrosis treated? 58
How is early avascular necrosis treated? 58
Is a core decompression a big operation? 59
What is the recovery after a core decompression? 59
If so few patients do well with a core decompression, then why is it done? 59
If hip replacements are so good, why would you want to avoid them in avascular necrosis in a young patient? 59
If a core decompression does not relieve the pain in the hip in avascular necrosis, what is the next step? 60
How is late or advanced avascular necrosis treated? 60
Hip Infections **60**
What are the symptoms of a hip infection? 60
How is the diagnosis of a hip infection made? 60
What blood tests can help find out if there is a hip infection? 60
What x-ray type tests can help find out if there is a hip infection? 61
How is fluid removed from a hip joint to see if there is a hip infection? 61
What is an infection in a "native" hip? 61
What is a periprosthetic infection? 61
What is the recommended treatment of a native hip infection? .. 62
What eventually becomes of a joint that gets infected? 62
Can you replace a hip in a joint that was previously infected? 62
What is the recommended treatment of a hip replacement that becomes infected? 62
Treatment of children's Hip Problems that lead to Problems as Adults **63**
What type of doctor treats these children's hip problems? 63
How is developmental or congenital dysplasia of the hip DDH/CDH) treated? 63

What type of surgery is needed sometimes in DDH/CDH?...... 63
How is Legg-Calvé Perthes treated? 63
How is Slipped Capital Femoral Epiphysis (SCFE) treated?...... 64
What happens to patients with childhood hip problems when they reach adulthood?...... 64

Hip Fractures (Broken Hip) 64
What actually breaks in a hip fracture?...... 64
Why does a hip actually break? 64
What is osteoporosis?...... 64
How are hip fractures treated? 65
How is the treatment choice made in hip fractures?...... 65
What type of replacement is done for certain hip fractures? 66
After hip fracture surgery, what can a person expect?...... 66

Hip Tendonitis...... 67
What is hip tendonitis?...... 67
How is hip tendonitis treated? 67
Does hip tendonitis ever need surgery?...... 67

Hip Bursitis...... 67
How is hip bursitis treated? 67
Does hip bursitis ever need surgery?...... 68

Hip Replacement Surgery...... 69
What is a hip replacement? 70
How long have hip replacements been around? 70
What kind of doctor does hip replacements?...... 70
What type of company makes a hip replacement?...... 71
What are some of the more popular companies that make hip replacements? 71
Are there differences between companies and their models of hip replacements? 71
What are all the parts or components of a hip replacement?...... 71
What materials are a hip replacement made of?...... 72
What are the most common configurations hip replacements?... 73
What are other hip replacement configurations?...... 74
There are so many mixes and matches here- how is it decided what I get 75
Can you show me the difference of each configuratio? 75

If metal-on-metal is not as safe then why is it used?................ 75
How is the cup put in and fixed to the bone?........................... 76
How is the femoral component put in and fixed to the bone?....... 76
Do any of the parts wear out?... 76
If a polyethylene liner can wear out, then why don't surgeons use substitutes for polyethylene? 76
Can I request one type or another of configuration?................... 77
Who monitors the quality of these joint replacements?............... 77
What is the FDA?... 77
How do I know the product is safe?....................................... 77
Can I be allergic to a hip replacement?................................... 77
How is metal allergy tested? 78
I have heard about "recalls." What are these about?.................. 78
Who really chooses my joint replacement?.............................. 78
How do I know if I need A hip replacement?............................ 78
How do I "care" for a hip replacement to make it last longer?...... 79
What kind of activity specifically causes a hip replacement to wear out?... 79
In general, if I look at activity in three ways, low, medium, and high levels, then how long can a hip replacement last? 79
What is the average age of people who get hip replacements?.... 79
Is someone too young to get a hip replacement?...................... 80
Is someone too old to get a hip replacement? 80
Is someone too "sick" to get a hip replacement? 80
Is a hip replacement a "dangerous" operation?......................... 80
How long is the surgery? 80
Are there different surgical methods of replacing a hip? 81
What are the differences between these surgical approaches?.... 81
Which approach should I choose? 81
Can robots do this surgery?... 82
What are the surgical steps in a hip replacement?..................... 82
What are some of the complications? 86
What is a hip dislocation after hip replacement?....................... 86
Why does a hip dislocation happen and how is it prevented? 87
How does a leg length problem happen?................................. 87

9

How and when does a fracture (broken bone) occur in a hip replacement?... 88
How does a hip replacement loosen from Its attachment to the bone? 88
Why does a hip replacement get infected? 88
How is a total hip replacement infection diagnosed? 89
What is the treatment of an infected hip replacement? 89
How fast does it take to recover from a hip replacement? 89
How quickly can I get up out of bed and walk after surgery?......... 90
Can I go home after the surgery? 90
If I don't go home after the surgery, then where do I go? 90
How do I benefit from physical therapy? 90
How bad is the pain after the surgery?... 91
How is the pain relieved after surgery? 91
Aside from pain management, what other types of treatments are given to me after surgery? 91
Why is my blood thinned?.. 91
How do I choose a surgeon and what are his/her qualifications to do a hip replacement?... 92
Do you like the surgeon' general approach? 92
Did he/she take a thorough history and do a complete examination?.. 92
Did you like the way he/she explained all the steps? 92
Do you know where the surgeon trained?... 93
Did he/she do some type of joint replacement fellowship? 93
Does he/she do more than 25 hip replacements a year? 94
Is he/she board certified by the American Board of Orthopaedic Surgeons (ABOS)?... 94
Is he/she a member of the American Academy of Orthopaedic Surgeons? 94
Is he/she a member of The American Association of Hip and Knee Surgeons (AAHKS)?.. 94
Is the hospital a respected center?... 95
Does the surgeon have any publications in the field? 95
Does her/she lecture at meetings?... 95
Who pays for all the costs of joint replacement surgery? 95

Who actually pays for the joint replacement model itself? 95
How much does the hospital and the doctor actually get paid? ... 96
What are all the other parts of the surgery that cost money? 96
Are there any precautions after surgery that I need to worry about? 96
What about antibiotics for dental work and other procedures? .. 97
Will I trigger metal detectors? 97
How long is the hospital stay? 97
How do I decide to go to a rehabilitation facility or to home? 97
Do I get physical therapy after I get home? 97
What is the difference between physical therapy and occupational therapy? 98
What type of medical monitoring happens at home after surgery? 98
What kind of equipment do I have the option of having at home? 98
What activities can I do after a hip replacement? 99
What activities should I stay away from after a hip replacement? 99
When can I drive after a hip replacement? 99
When can I have sex after a hip replacement? 99
What is revision hip surgery? 100
When is hip revision surgery necessary? 100
How successful is hip surgery a second or third time? 100
Do I need to see a medical doctor before the surgery? 100
What is an anesthesiologist? 100
What kind of anesthesia do I get for hip replacement surgery? .101
What is general anesthesia? 101
What is spinal anesthesia? 101
What is regional anesthesia? 101
Can you give me a summary of what happens, hour-by-hour and day-by-day after the surgery? 102
Will I need a transfusion after a hip replacement? 102
What are the signs that a hip replacement is starting to fail? 102
When are the stitches or staples removed after surgery? 103
How often will I see my doctor after surgery? 103

Surface Replacements, Hip Arthroscopy, Labrum Tears, and Femoroacetabular impingement 104

    What is a surface replacement? 105
    How long have surface replacements been around? 105
    Why would some surgeons recommend a surface replacement? 105
    Is a hip resurfacing less invasive than a total hip replacement? 105
    Is there any specific reason not to have a hip resurfacing? 107
    When would someone recommend a surface replacement instead of a hip replacement? 107
    What is hip arthroscopy? 108
    What types of disorders does hip arthroscopy treat? 108
    Can hip arthroscopy be used to treat arthritis? 109
    Is hip arthroscopy successful for the other problems beside arthritis, FAI, and labrum tears? 109

Common questions about some practical issues about surgery 110

    What happens on the first appointment? 111
    what are the steps leading up to surgery? 111
    I already have my own medical doctor. Why would my surgeon send me to a medical doctor in their center?? 111
    What specific tests are done before the surgery? 112
    Are there any other doctors I will have to see before the surgery? 113
    Do I see the Anesthesiologist prior to surgery? 113
    What arrangements do I need to make prior to the surgery? 113
    What general medical instructions do I need to follow starting the week before surgery? 114
    What general instructions do I follow the day before surgery? . 114
    What time do I get to the hospital on the day of surgery? 115
    Once I get to the hospital how long do I wait until the surgery? 115
    After the surgery is over, where do I go after the operating room? 115
    When can my family of friends visit me? 115
    What can I expect in the first 24 hours after surgery? 116

How is my pain treated? 116
What will the next few days look like? 116
After I go to a rehabilitation home or to my own home, when do I come back to see my surgeon? 116
How often do I have physical therapy after I get discharged from the hospital? 117
What specific things should I worry about after I get home? 117
What if I have questions after I leave the hospital? 117

A few final statements from the author 118

INTRODUCTION

WHAT IS THIS BOOK ABOUT?

Many people have pain in their body. Sometimes that pain is in your joints. This book is about that pain. When you read this book you will learn why you have pain in your joints and about the many ways you can get rid of that pain.

HOW DO I READ THIS BOOK?

This book is not meant to be read from the beginning to the end. It is organized by questions. I wrote it this way because after over twenty years of treating patients with joint problems, I learned as much from patients asking me questions as they did by my answering them. You can open up any page of this book and start reading and learning.

WHAT IF I HAVE MORE QUESTIONS?

Of course you can go on the Internet and search these terms but the amount of information you encounter will be huge. I have a better idea. Go on the Internet and send me a question. My website is:

www.irathek.com

There is a big button ASK A QUESTION

When you ask it we will answer it and then possibly include it in the next version of the book!

WHY DID YOU WRITE THIS BOOK?

I wrote it because there were so many patients who came into the office who asked great questions. This led me to believe that the educational material we were giving patients was simply not answering all the questions they had. I always felt that a question/answer format is easy to read and also is effective.

GENERAL QUESTIONS ABOUT JOINTS

WHY DOES SOMEONE HAVE JOINT PAIN?

We really don't know the answer to that all the time. There are some obvious reasons we can discuss. If you twist a joint you can tear some of the supporting structures of the joint. When you tear these things, the body responds by sending all kinds of cells and chemicals to the site. The cells and chemicals produce other chemicals that literally cause pain. The actual process of why one person feels more pain and others feel less with the same problem is poorly understood.

WHAT ARE SOME OF THE MORE COMMON CONDITIONS THAT CAUSE JOINT PAIN?

Joint pains can come from a number of reasons. Here is a table that summarizes the major ones:

Injury	A fall or an accident can cause a broken bone that can involve the surface of the joint. Over time the joint gets destroyed.
Age	As some people age, the cartilage surface simply wears out. This is called osteoarthritis.
Inflammation	Some arthritis like gout, rheumatoid arthritis, and Lyme disease can cause the body to produce chemicals that can inflame the covering or lining of the joint
Infection	A bacterial infection can destroy the cartilage rapidly.

WHAT EXACTLY IS A JOINT IN THE BODY?

A joint is a space between two or more bones. In the body there are many joints.

DO ALL JOINTS MOVE?

No. Some joints move like the knee joint and the shoulder joint. There are many joints that barely have any movement at all. More commonly these are joints in the spine and the wrist and the foot.

THAT DOESN'T MAKE SENSE TO ME. HOW DOES A JOINT NOT MOVE?

Imagine a table in your kitchen. It has a tabletop and legs. The legs are connected to the top by joints. These joints don't move. They are rigid joints. In the body, there are joints in the spine, hand, and foot that have very little motion and don't move like we think of joints moving. These joints really don't move but sort of rub over each other as they connect one bone to another.

DOES IT MATTER WHETHER SOME JOINTS MOVE AND SOME JOINTS DON'T MOVE?

Joints are a source of pain when they are injured, aged, inflamed or infected. It doesn't matter whether they move or not. Joints that move tend to be more painful when they move, though.

WHAT TYPES OF JOINTS ARE THERE IN THE BODY?

The are a few types of joints-

1. Ball and socket
2. Hinge and mortise-tenon
3. Side-to-side (non-moveable)

WHAT TYPE OF JOINT IS A HIP JOINT?

The hip joint is a deep ball and socket joint

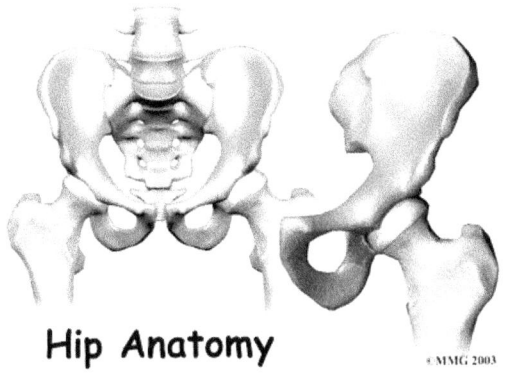

Hip Anatomy

WHAT TYPE OF JOINT IS THE KNEE JOINT?

It is a hinge joint.

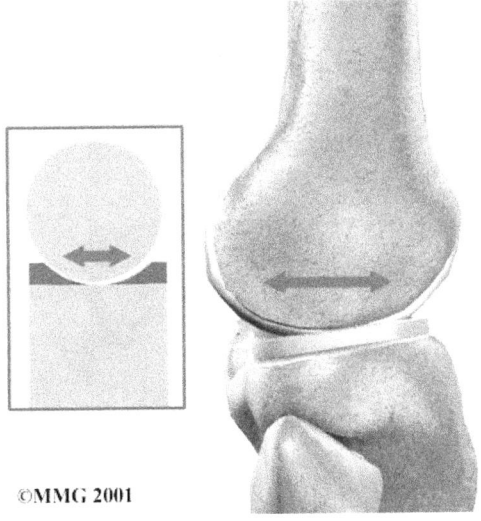

The knee joint

WHAT TYPE OF JOINT IS THE SHOULDER JOINT?

The shoulder joint is a shallow ball and socket joint.

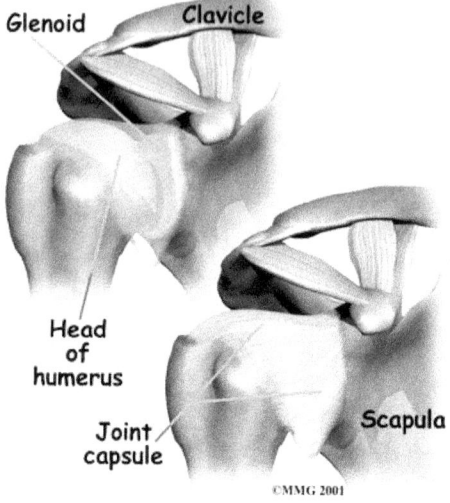

WHAT TYPE OF JOINT IS THE ELBOW JOINT?

The elbow has two joints- a ball and socket part and a hinge part.

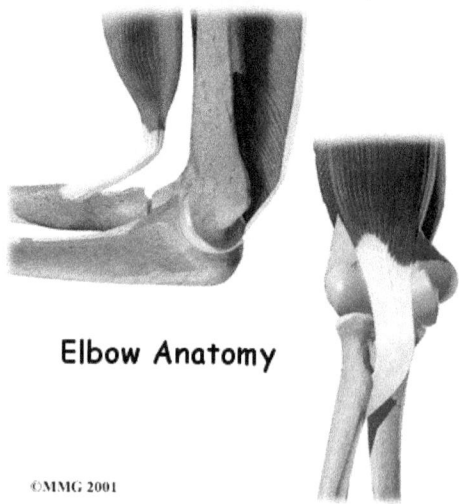

Elbow Anatomy

WHAT TYPE OF JOINT IS THE WRIST AND HAND JOINTS?

The wrist joint is a hinge joint in one part but there are also non-moveable joints in the wrist. The fingers have hinge joints.

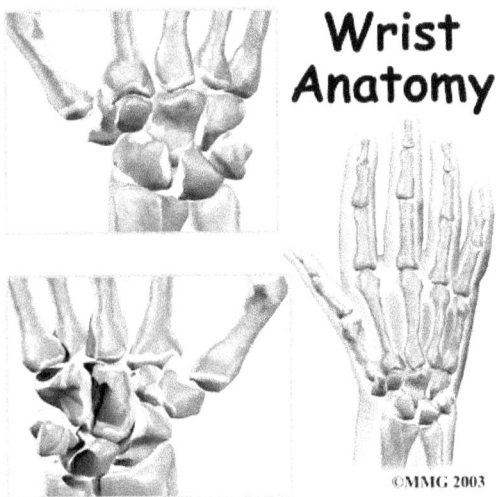

WHAT TYPE OF JOINT IS THE ANKLE JOINT?

The ankle is a special joint called a mortise and tenon joint. This is similar to a leg on a table. The table leg (tenon) goes into a hole in the table top (mortise). In the ankle, the talus (tenon) goes into a space make by the tibia and the fibula (mortise).

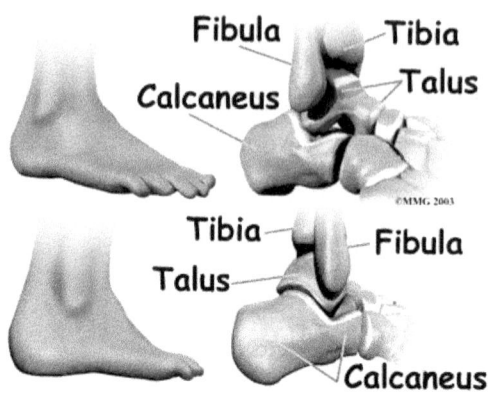

The ankle joint is made up of three bones

WHAT TYPES OF JOINTS ARE IN THE FOOT?

The midfoot mainly has side-to-side joints that barely move. The toes are hinge joints.

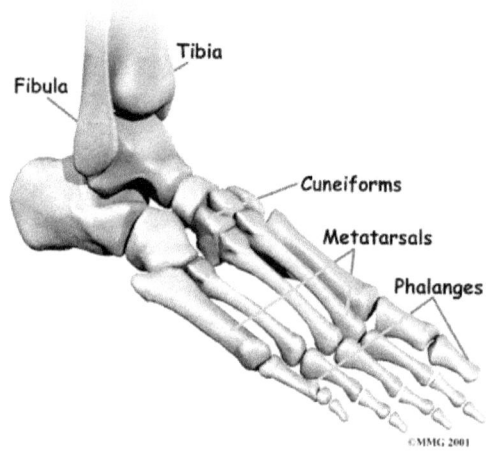

The foot has a rigid midfoot and a flexible forefoot

WHAT MAKES JOINTS SO SMOOTH AND CUSHIONY?

Cartilage. The ends of each bone that form a joint are covered with cartilage. Cartilage is a very strong, smooth, and cushiony surface. It feels like greasy rubber and functions that way.

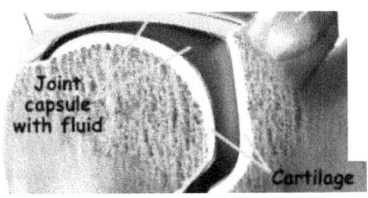

Cartilage covers the end of bones at the joint

I HAVE HEARD ABOUT JOINT LUBRICATION. IS THERE REALLY SUCH A THING?

Yes and no. Within every joint there is a thick, greasy fluid called synovial fluid. We commonly call it joint fluid. Joint fluid does allow for some lubrication, but it also supplies nutrition for the cartilage.

WHERE DOES JOINT FLUID COME FROM?

The lining of the joint makes joint fluid. All joints are surrounded by a lining or capsule type structure that has nutritional cells on the inside layer (synovial cells) that produce fluid. The fluid gives cartilage its nutrition because cartilage does not have a good blood supply. Joints also have a thicker outer layer that gives mechanical support to the joint.

WHY DOES CARTILAGE LOSE ITS EFFECTIVENESS?

The four reasons that give you joint pain also contribute to cartilage effectiveness: Infection, inflammation, Injury, Age. All of these can cause cartilage thinning, softening, or degeneration (destruction).

WHAT DOES INFECTION DO TO THE CARTILAGE AND THE JOINT?

Infection is one of the worst attacks to a joint. Infections sometimes are so bad that the joint is nearly completely destroyed within days. Other infections are not as bad. The bacteria essentially eat away at the cartilage.

WHAT DOES INFLAMMATION DO TO THE CARTILAGE AND THE JOINT?

Joint inflammation like rheumatoid arthritis or gout produces white cells that produce chemicals that first cause joint pain without cartilage destruction. Over time, if it persists, the inflammation eventually invades the cartilage itself and causes it to get destroyed.

WHAT DOES AN INJURY DO TO THE CARTILAGE AND THE JOINT?

If a broken bone extends into the joint, the cartilage cells can get directly crushed and they can't recover from that because cartilage cells do not repair themselves (they do not regenerate). The cartilage-cartilage joint surface needs to be smooth on both sides. If a break splits one side open then the surface is no longer smooth unless it is screwed together by an operation.

WHAT DOES AGING DO TO THE CARTILAGE AND THE JOINT?

We are not sure how this happens, but over time, in some people, the cartilage cells start to die or lose their strength to support the joint. This is called cartilage degeneration. The term osteoarthritis is commonly used for this type of joint degeneration. When this happens the smooth surface of the cartilage starts to get rougher. Eventually it wears completely away down to the bone surface.

WHAT IS ARTHRITIS?

Arthritis is pain because of some problem with the joint lining or destruction of the cartilage of a joint.

HOW DO I KNOW A JOINT HAS ARTHRITIS?

You don't unless you've had an x-ray or another type of test. Sometimes joint pain can be a side effect of medications you are taking so it really is not arthritis. X-ray, MRI, and CT scan are common tests to decide whether you have arthritis.

WHAT ARE THE DIFFERENCES BETWEEN AN X-RAY, MRI, AND CT SCAN?

An x-ray is a test that uses radiation to take a picture of things in your body that have different amounts of density. You can bone but you can see cartilage, blood vessels, or fluid. It is a good test for basic arthritis. An MRI (magnetic resonance imaging) is a magnetic test, without radiation, that can see bone, cartilage, tendons, ligaments, and fluid. It provides a lot of information. In arthritis, though, most information comes from a basic x-ray. You can do x-rays while the patient is standing which shows how well the cartilage supports the joint. Certain diseases need an MRI to make the diagnosis. A CT scan is a test using a lot of radiation that can show excellent bone detail. You also can develop 3D pictures using a CT scan.

ARE THERE DIFFERENT DEGREES OF CARTILAGE LOSS OR IS IT THERE ONE DAY AND GONE THE NEXT?

Arthritis has many looks. To make it easy I will say that it is mild, moderate, or severe. Let's use as an example your kitchen floor. Let's say that the floor originally was wood and you decided to put a layer of shiny tile on top. The shiny, smooth surface of this tile is the cartilage and the wood underneath is your bone. The tile starts off

1/4 inch thick. Over time, with your family walking on the tile the surface begins to dull and wear. It is still ¼ inch thick but is no longer as smooth. This is mild arthritis. Over more time, with more wear the 1/4 tile wears down in sections to 1/8 inch. This is moderate arthritis. Then eventually some areas wear all the way down to the wood (your bone). This is severe arthritis.

WHAT DOES AN X-RAY SHOW IN ARTHRITIS?

X-rays only show bone. The space between two bones is filled with cartilage. Therefore an x-ray will show this space in a normal joint but in a joint with arthritis there will be no space seen. This is why we sometimes call this bone-on-bone arthritis.

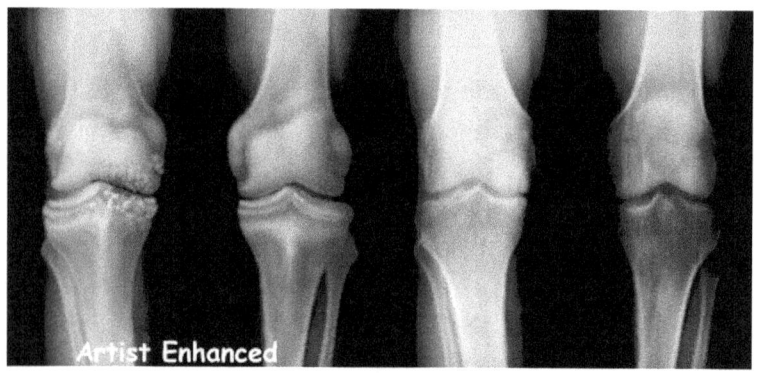

Arthritis is seen as bone-on-bone on an x-ray

WHAT ARE SOME OF THE OTHER WAYS TO FIND OUT WHAT TYPE OF JOINT PROBLEM I HAVE?

Sometimes an x-ray is normal but a laboratory blood test can show you have an inflammation causing the arthritis such as rheumatoid arthritis or gout. Rheumatoid arthritis is a disease where the body produces inflammation cells that build up around joint. Gout is a problem where the body produces tiny crystals that fill up joints. Sometimes we can remove joint fluid and look under a microscope to tell you why you have arthritis. Other times an MRI (magnetic resonance imaging) can see arthritis when an x-ray can't. An MRI is a test where you can see the cartilage surface.

WHAT ARE SOME OF THE GENERAL WAYS TO TREAT JOINT PROBLEMS?

So much depends on the actual joint but in general, the there are a few ways to look at treatment of the joint.

- The "Who is Treating My Joint" Approach to Joint Pain Treatment
    Either you are treating yourself, or a doctor or physical therapist is advising you what to do.

- The "What is Going Into My Body" Approach to Joint Pain Treatment
    You can take pills, rub creams, or get injections to treat the joint. Injections can be either into blood, skin, or the joint itself.

- The "Someone Touches My Body Approach"
    You can work with a trainer to do exercise, a physical therapist to do prescribed treatment, or you can get surgery.

WHEN YOU SAY I CAN TREAT MYSELF, WHAT DOES THAT MEAN?

We often do things to help ourselves. We can put ice on an injured joint. We can rest it. We can use a cane or a walking stick. We can even go to the pharmacy and buy simple pain relievers such as Tylenol (acetaminophen) or Advil, Motrin (ibuprofen), or Aleve (naproxyn).

WHAT ARE THE COMMON TYPES OF PRESCRIPTION MEDICINES I TAKE FOR ARTHRITIS"?

Doctors can prescribe prescription strengths of the drugs you can take on your own that may be stronger. Sometime you can take narcotic pain relievers such as hydrocodone (Vicodan), and oxycodone (Percocet). Doctors can also inject medicine like cortisone into the joint. For certain types of arthritis, such as rheumatoid, there are medicines that are injected that can slow this disease. These are injected into the bloodstream. Some common brand names are Enbrel and Remicade.

DO EXERCISE AND PHYSICAL THERAPY WORK FOR ARTHRITIS?

It really depends on the specific joint. Most joints respond well to exercise and physical therapy. Not all joints are helped by physical therapy. Sometimes, when the arthritis is so bad, any movement can hurt too much.

DOES MY WEIGHT HAVE ANYTHING TO DO WITH ARTHRITIS OR JOINT PAIN?

In general, joints that see your weight are the spine, hip, knee, ankle, and foot. While no one really knows whether being overweight causes the arthritis to get worse, it is probably true that the pain from arthritis is worse when you are overweight.

WHAT TYPES OF DOCTORS TREAT WHICH TYPES OF JOINT PROBLEMS?

Your general medical or family doctor can treat most types of joint pain. Sometimes, if you have a special form of arthritis like rheumatoid arthritis a rheumatologist may treat you. This is a doctor who trained in the field of Internal Medicine and then did extra training in joint diseases. A rheumatologist uses non-surgical methods. Another type of health professional that treats arthritis is a chiropractor who manipulates and realigns joints to decrease pain. For the foot, podiatrists can do non-surgical and surgical treatments. Orthopaedists or orthopaedic Surgeons do non-surgical and surgical treatment of all joints. It is very common to have more than one of these specialists involved in your care. They often work together in your best interests.

GENERAL QUESTIONS ABOUT THE HIP

WHAT AND WHERE IS THE HIP JOINT?

The hip joint connects your pelvic bone to your legs. It is a large and strong joint. As you can see from the picture, it is a ball and socket joint. The hip joint has a deep socket and a large ball. The socket is sometimes called the cup. The leg bone that the pelvic bone connects to is called the femur. The ball that connects to the socket of cup is called the head of the femur. Since the cup is so deep, the hip is a very stable joint. It very rarely "pops out" of the joint. The pronunciation of these medical words is as follows:

Femur is pronounced: fee-mer
Acetabulum is pronounced: a-se-ta-bew-lum

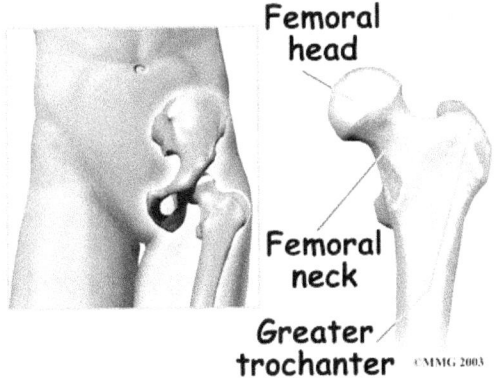

The hip joint itself in near the groin

ARE THERE OTHER THINGS BESIDES THE CUP AND BALL THAT ARE PART OF THE HIP JOINT?

Yes. There is the labrum, ligaments, muscles, tendons, and bursa.

WHAT IS THE LABRUM?

The hip cup has a ring around it. It is called the labrum. Since the cup is called the acetabulum, the labrum is called the acetabular labrum. It is like a gasket that is around a faucet. While you can imagine it sort of "seals" the joint, it actually is more involved in giving the joint a little more stability. The ring of the labrum stabilizes the joint at the edges of the cup.

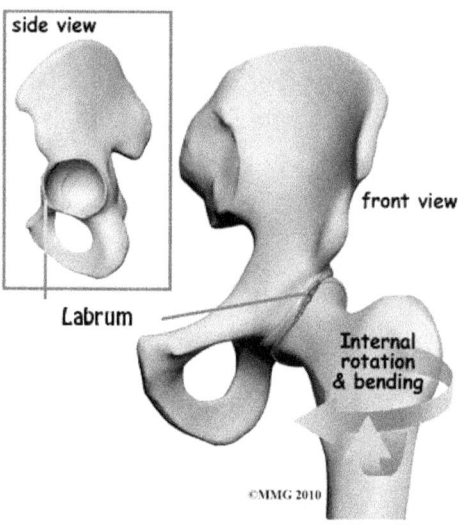

The labrum helps support the ball in the socket

ARE HIP LIGAMENTS IMPORTANT?

Yes. Ligaments are ropes that connect one bone to another bone and give it stability. Stability in the hip means that when you move the hip it does not pop out of the joint and wiggle around too much.

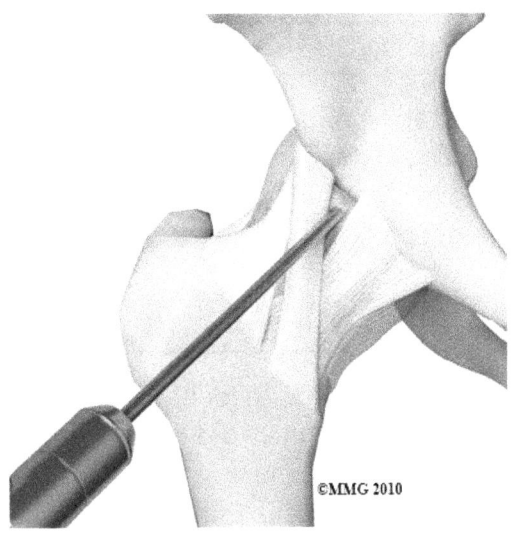

The ligaments are the white crisscross structures

WHAT DO THE MUSCLES AROUND THE HIP JOINT DO?

The muscles actually move one bone over another. There are many muscles and they all work together to allow you to do all types of hip movements smoothly and with enough strength.

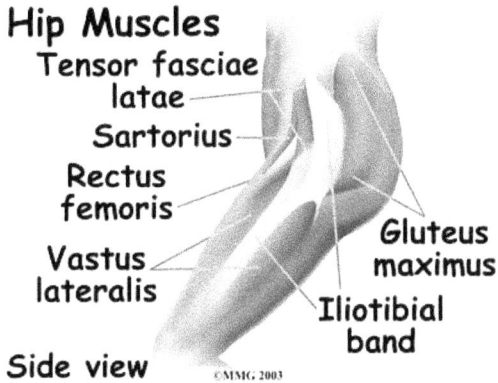

There are many muscles around the hip joint

WHAT ARE THE TENDONS AROUND THE HIP JOINT?

Tendons are tight ropes at the end of muscle. They are the connectors of the muscles to the bone. Sometimes they are too tight or too loose and other times they get irritated or inflamed and are a reason you can get pain. This is called tendonitis.

WHAT IS THE HIP BURSA?

A bursa is a greasy film that protects tendons from rough edges of bone. A lot of joints have bursae (the word bursae is the plural of bursa). The hip bursa is located along the outside of the hip joint in an area you can actually feel yourself. Sometimes this bursa gets inflamed and is a source of pain.

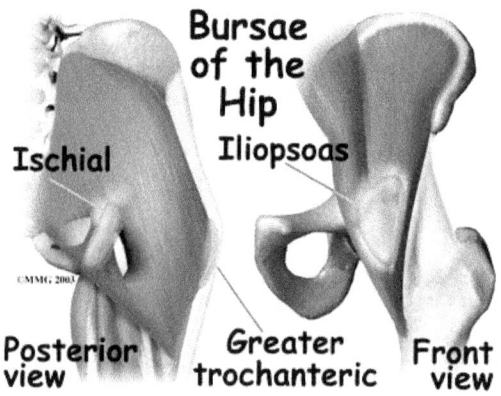

There are two bursae around the hip joint

IF I WERE STANDING AND LOOKING AT MYSELF IN THE MIRROR AND WANTED TO POINT TO MY HIP JOINTS, WHERE WOULD THEY BE?

The actual joint itself is near the groin. I answer this question because many times people come to the office and say they are complaining of "hip" pain but actually point to the lower and side part of the back. Hip joint pain is actually in the groin.

WHAT ARE THE MORE COMMON PROBLEMS THAT CAUSE PAIN IN THE HIP JOINT?

The hip joint most commonly has the following problems:

1. Arthritis
2. Bursitis
3. Fracture
4. Labrum tear
5. Impingement

WHAT IS ARTHRITIS OF THE HIP?

Arthritis of the hip joint is when the soft cartilage surface of the acetabulum (socket of cup) and the femoral head (ball) is worn out, has holes in it, or is destroyed. Essentially, instead of having a cushion there, there is bone rubbing against bone.

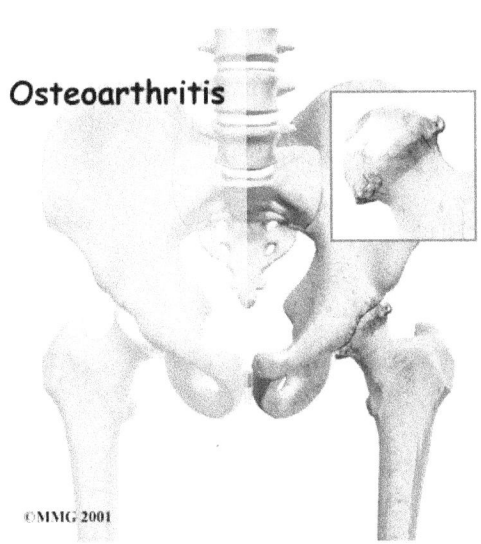

Arthritis can destroy the cartilage surfaces of a joint

WHAT CAUSES ARTHRITIS OF THE HIP?

Some types of arthritis have a cause and others do not. The most common form of arthritis is called osteoarthritis and this is usually thought of as an age-related wear and tear of the cartilage surface. The cause is not known. It just seems to happen. You don't inherit osteoarthritis from your parents but some people think that the risk of developing osteoarthritis is increased in some families.

A second kind of arthritis is rheumatoid arthritis. This is a problem with the lining around the joints. In rheumatoid arthritis the lining produces cells that make inflammatory chemicals that then destroy the joint.

A third kind of arthritis is arthritis from an injury. Doctors often use the word "trauma" to substitute for the word injury. A car accident or a fall from a height can produce an injury to the hip by either causing a crush of the cartilage surface or a break in the bone that goes all the way into the hip joint surface. Months or even years after a trauma to the hip joint, arthritis can develop. We call this post-traumatic arthritis. The word "post" means "after." Therefore, post-traumatic arthritis means arthritis after a trauma.

A fourth type of arthritis is joint destruction from an infection. Bacteria (and not viruses) can destroy the cartilage surface. Sometimes the joint can be destroyed in just a few days with certain types of very bad infections.

A fifth type of arthritis is one that develops because the person had a problem with their hips when they were children. Later in life this problem can lead to arthritis.

WHAT TYPE OF HIP PROBLEMS IN CHILDREN CAN LEAD TO HIP ARTHRITIS AS AN ADULT?

There are three common childhood hip problems that can cause arthritis in adulthood. These are developmental dysplasia, slipped capital femoral epiphysis, and Legg-Calvé-Perthes disease.

WHAT IS DEVELOPMENTAL DYSPLASIA OF THE HIP?

This is a problem that occurs in the first few years of life. It can start as early as a few weeks after birth up to a few years. It is a problem where the hip joint either does not develop correctly as a round ball and socket or in the worst cases, does not develop at all. There are many treatments for this problem but even with treatment, many of these people will get arthritis at a younger age (as young as in their 20's and 30's).

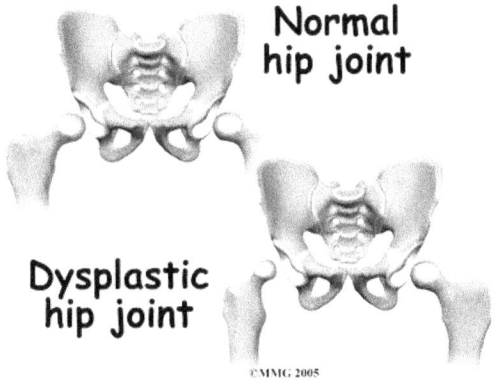

The hip is not formed completely in a dysplastic joint

WHAT IS LEGG-CALVÉ-PERTHES DISEASE OF THE HIP?

This is a problem that occurs in children ages 5-10 when the blood supply to the hip joins can get interrupted. This can cause the ball of the hip joint to have areas that literally die. There is treatment but some of these patients develop hip arthritis early- as young as in their 30's or 40's. The reason it is called Legg-Calvé-Perthes is because those were the names of the doctors who described this condition- Dr. Legg, Dr. Calvé, and Dr. Perthes. Sometimes doctors just refer to this problem as Perthes disease.

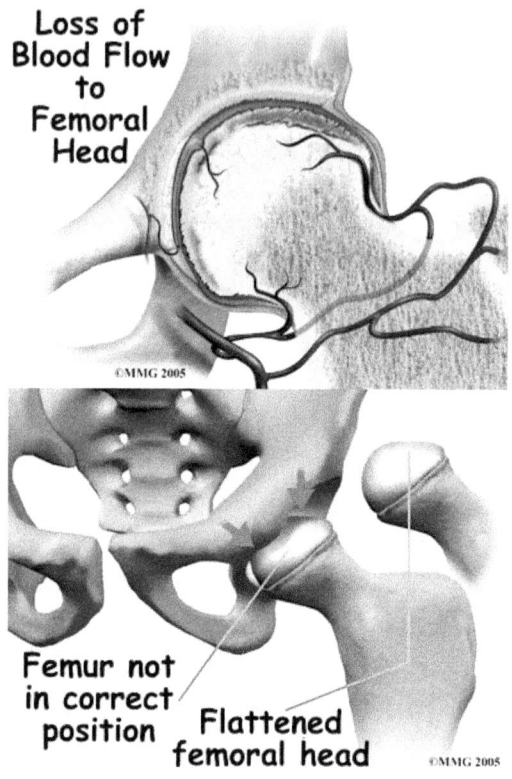

The loss of blood supply causes flattening of the femoral head in Legg-Calvé-Perthes

WHAT IS SLIPPED CAPITAL FEMORAL EPIPHYSIS OF THE HIP?

This is a problem that affects children ages 12-16. The ball of the hip joint has a growth plate that in some people can slip off its base. This usually needs surgery to prevent further slipping or to put the slip back in place. Some of the people who had this problem develop arthritis at a younger age- most commonly in their 40's and 50's.

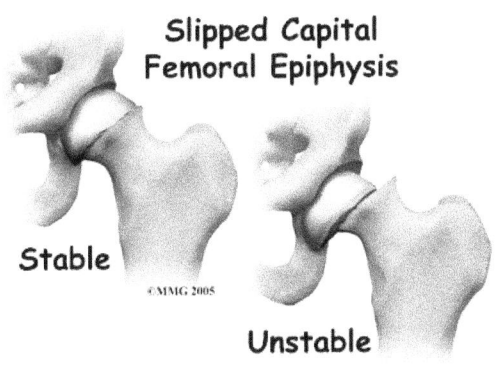

The femoral head literally slips off in a slipped capital femoral epiphysis

AT WHAT AGE DOES HIP ARTHRITIS AFFECT PEOPLE?

Except for the child hip problems discussed in the last few questions (which generally are not common anyway), most arthritis of the hip starts when a person is in their 40's and gets more common as they get older. Depending on the part of the world and the community, the 60's and 70-'s are the most common ages for arthritis of the hip joint that needs treatment.

WHAT DOES AN X-RAY OF ARTHRITIS OF THE HIP JOINT LOOK LIKE?

A normal x-ray of a hip shows a nice space between the ball and socket joint. That space is actually filled with cartilage. Cartilage cannot be seen on an x-ray so it looks like a space. When the cartilage is worn down it becomes thinner and the space gets smaller. Eventually, when the arthritis is severe and there is no cartilage, there is no space at all.

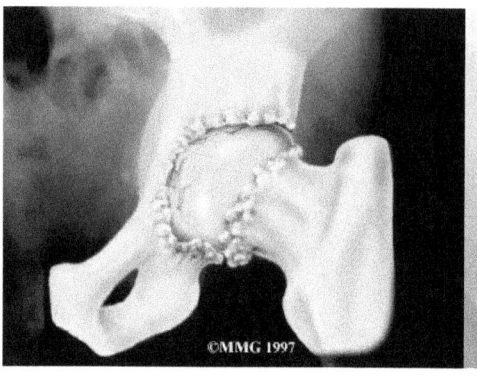
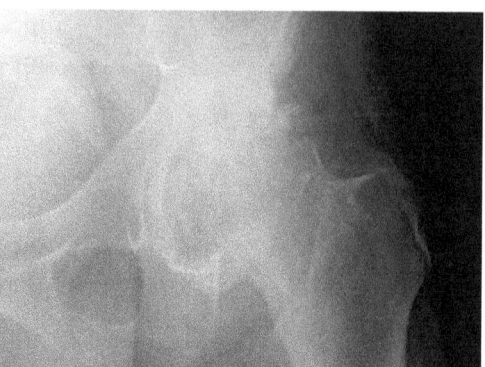

Arthritis can be very destructive of the joint surface

WHAT IS A FRACTURE OR A BROKEN HIP?

Fractures are broken bones, so a fracture of the hip literally is a break in different areas of the hip joint.

WHAT DOES AN X-RAY OF A FRACTURE OR A BROKEN HIP OF THE HIP JOINT LOOK LIKE?

The x-ray is the best way to see a fracture or break and it shows exactly where the hip fracture is and how severe it is.

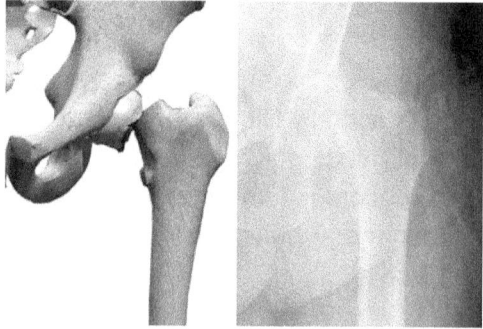

The bone often completely breaks through in a hip fracture

WHAT ARE OTHER PROBLEMS OF THE HIP JOINT?

The other most common problems of the hip joint are avascular necrosis, hip bursitis, labrum tear, hip impingement, and hip infection

WHAT IS AVASCULAR NECROSIS?

Avascular necrosis of the hip is a problem of the blood supply that goes to the ball of the hip (the ball is the head of the femur). It is sometimes called "aseptic necrosis." The word "aseptic" means not infected. The word "septic" means infected. For reasons that are not completely understood, the blood supply gets blocked and the bone in the joint begins to die. In fact, the word "necrosis of the bone" means "death of the bone." When the bone dies, the cartilage surface gets destroyed and the smooth joint surface is now collapsed and rough.

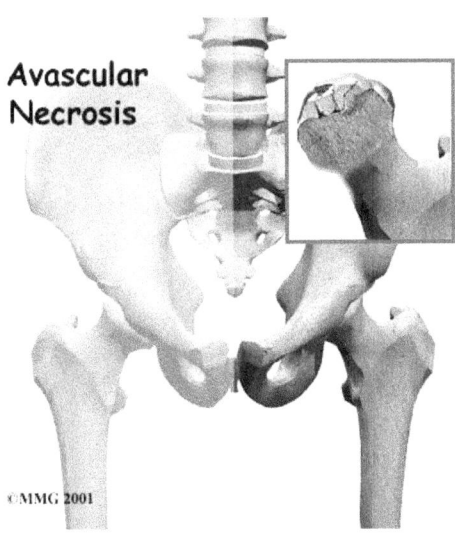

Avascular necrosis can cause serious destruction of the hip joint

WHAT CAUSES AVASCULAR NECROSIS?

While we don't know exactly what causes the disruption of the blood supply, we know that certain things increase a person's risk of developing avascular necrosis and the most common of these include a previous fracture (break) of the hip, oral steroid medications (like asthma steroids), alcoholism, and sickle cell anemia.

WHAT IS HIP BURSITIS?

Hip bursitis is an inflammation of the bursa of the hip. There are two common bursae- the bursa on the outer side of the hip called the trochanteric bursa and the bursa in the area of where you sit (your buttock) called the ischial bursa. The bursae in these areas protect certain tendons from the bone.

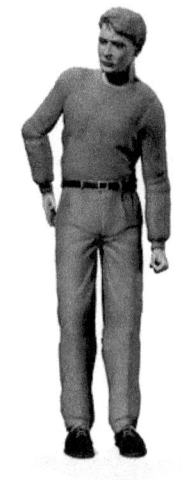

Pain area in trochanteric bursitis

Patients often limp when they have trochanteric bursitis

WHAT CAUSES HIP BURSITIS?

Hip bursitis is usually caused by: (1) a direct injury to the bursa such as a fall or a punch, (2) age-related degeneration of the bursa, or (3) overuse.

WHAT IS A LABRUM TEAR?

The hip labrum is the cartilage ring that is around the acetabulum. As noted earlier, it is like a rubber gasket that seals a faucet. The labrum is involved in hip stability. While it really does not "seal" the joint, it functions to assist the ligaments to keep the hip stable in the socket. A tear in a labrum is either an actual cut in the ring or when the attachment of the ring to the bone is disrupted.

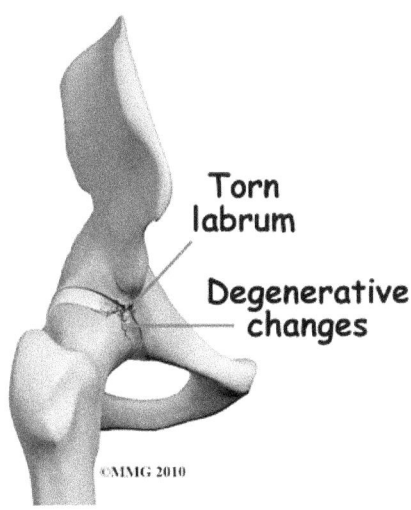

When the labrum tears it can be very painful

WHAT IS HIP IMPINGEMENT OR FEMOROACETABULAR IMPINGEMENT?

Hip impingement is an early form of arthritis that is restricted to a small area of the outer portion of the hip joint. It is important to recognize this as different from other forms of arthritis because it may be possible to treat this with less invasive operations.

HOW IMPORTANT IS IT FOR ME TO ACTUALLY KNOW WHY I HAVE HIP PAIN?

The treatment is different depending upon what type of hip arthritis you have so it is important to know your diagnosis or underlying cause.

TREATMENT OF SPECIFIC HIP PROBLEMS

HIP ARTHRITIS

WHAT ARE SOME OF THE NON-SURGICAL TREATMENTS OF HIP ARTHRITIS?

Hip arthritis can be treated by changing your activities, using a cane or something similar when walking, prescription medications, non-prescription medications, nutritional supplements, injections, and physical therapy.

DO ANY OF THESE TREATMENTS REVERSE ARTHRITIS OR BUILD CARTILAGE?

No. If they work at all, they work to decrease the pain. There is nothing we know of that heals, builds, or physically adds support to the actual cartilage surface.

HOW DO I CHANGE MY ACTIVITY LEVEL TO HELP MY HIP ARTHRITIS?

This is the simplest way to help with your pain. If you normally jog 5 miles, try 3. If you play singles tennis or handball, play doubles. Take more elevators than stairs. All this helps with the pain. It also helps to wear soft-soled shoes.

DOES USING A CANE ACTUALLY WORK?

A cane in the hand opposite to your hip arthritis is a great way to decrease the pain while walking. There are many scientific studies that a cane used this way actually decreases the force across the hip joint. Less force equals less pain.

WHAT ARE ANTI-INFLAMMATORY MEDICATIONS?

There are three types of drugs that decrease inflammation and treat arthritis, tumor necrosis factors (TNFs), steroids and non-steroidal anti-inflammatory drugs (NSAIDS).

WHAT ARE TUMOR NECROSIS FACTORS (TNFS)?

TNFs are powerful drugs, given by injection into the bloodstream, that specifically treat rheumatoid arthritis. Two common TNFs are Enbrel and Remicade.

WHAT ARE STEROIDS?

Steroids are powerful drugs that attack inflammation whether they are given by mouth or injected into the joint.

ARE ANTI-INFLAMMATORY STEROIDS THE SAME AS THE STEROIDS WE HEAR ABOUT THAT ATHLETES TAKE TO IMPROVE PERFORMANCE?

No. The athletes take a very different form of steroids called "anabolic steroids." These are designed to build muscle and strength and do not fight inflammation.

HOW ARE STEROIDS GIVEN?

By mouth (oral) or injection.

WHAT ARE SOME OF THE NAMES OF VARIOUS ANTI-INFLAMMATORY STEROIDS?

Prednisone, triamcinolone or Kenalog, Depo-medrol, dexamethasone, Celestone.

WHAT ARE THE DIFFERENCES BETWEEN ALL THESE BRANDS OF STEROIDS?

They usually differ in how they are absorbed or other chemical differences that don't really make a big difference to each patient.

WHAT ARE THE POSITIVES ABOUT STEROIDS BY MOUTH?

Oral steroids are really amazing anti-inflammatory medications. They are the strongest anti-inflammatory medications you can get. They not only work well, they work fast.

WHAT ARE THE NEGATIVES ABOUT STEROIDS BY MOUTH?

Unfortunately there are a lot of side effects with oral steroids. They make you feel bloated by retaining water throughout your body. They weaken the strength of bone. They cause fat to develop in your liver. They lower your immune system. They can cause a loss of blood supply (avascular necrosis) to certain joints.

IF THERE ARE SO MANY NEGATIVES ABOUT ORAL STEROIDS, THEN WHY EVEN TAKE THEM?

The side effects are mainly a problem when you take steroids for longer periods of time. It is rare for these side effects to happen when you take steroids for a short time. You need to be under careful supervision from a doctor when you take steroids.

WHAT ARE THE POSITIVES ABOUT STEROID INJECTIONS INTO JOINTS?

When steroids can be injected directly into the inflamed joint there are two advantages. The first is that the powerful effect of the steroid is concentrated in the joint. When you take the steroid by mouth, the drug goes all over the body. When you inject it most of the medicine stays in the joint. The second is that by mainly staying in the joint, it does not circulate to the rest of the body. This means that injected steroid can have less side effects to other parts of your body.

WHAT ARE THE NEGATIVES ABOUT STEROID INJECTIONS?

There are a few negatives about steroid injections in and around joints. If some of the steroid is injected in a tendon it can weaken the tendon and cause it to rupture. Too many injections can also weaken the ligaments around a joint. Diabetics have to be especially careful because joint injections can raise a person's glucose (sugar) level rapidly.

WHAT TYPE OF INJECTIONS CAN I GET FOR HIP ARTHRITIS?

First of all, steroid injections are not commonly given for hip arthritis. The reason is that it is not an easy joint to reach with an injection. In an office a knee joint injection is simple but a hip joint usually needs to be done with some sort of x-ray or other type of radiology guidance (like CT scan or ultrasound). This makes it more cumbersome and expensive.

HOW DOES A CORTISONE INJECTION WORK?

The cortisone directly decreases the inflammatory cells that surround the joint.

IS THERE A LIMIT TO THE NUMBER OF CORTISONE INJECTIONS I CAN GET?

While there is no real rule here, most doctors talk about no more than 2-3 injections a year. Many doctors feel that too much cortisone in the joint will make the ligaments and tendons too weak. Also, if you need that many injections, then the steroid is probably not working well so there is no reason to continue. The only possible exception to this is people who are definitely getting benefit from injections every 3-4 months and for medical reasons cannot get any other treatment such as surgery.

WHAT IS A HYALURONIC ACID INJECTION?

Hyaluronic acid in a person's body is actually the main part of the fluid (synovial fluid) that lubricates and feeds the joint surface. Some companies have made synthetic hyaluronic acid from different sources such as rooster cartilage. It is packaged sterilely for injection. Some of the common names are Synvisc, Hyalgan, OrthoVisc, and Euflexxa.

HOW DO HYALURONIC ACID INJECTIONS WORK FOR ARTHRITIS OF THE HIP?

We are really not totally sure about how these injections work. In general, we can say that some patients definitely receive pain relief and increase joint flexibility for many months after an injection.

DOES HYALURONIC ACID BUILD CARTILAGE?

No.

IS THERE A LIMIT TO THE NUMBER OF HYALURONIC ACID INJECTIONS I CAN GET FOR ARTHRITIS OF THE HIP?

Unlike steroid injections it is generally believed there is no limit to the number of these injections over time but there have not been a lot of studies to answer this question.

WHAT ARE NSAIDS?

NSAIDS refer to Non-Steroidal Anti-Inflammatory Drugs. This is pronounced "en-sades." These are very common both with and without a prescription. Common NSAIDS are ibuprofen (Advil, Motrin), naproxen (Aleve, Naprosyn), meloxicam (Mobic)), diclofenac (Voltaren), sulindac (Clinoril), celecoxib (Celebrex), nambutone (Relafen), and indomethacin (Indocin).

HOW DO NSAIDS ACTUALLY WORK?

They are chemicals that interfere with the body's ability to produce inflammation. Inflammation is often a source of pain in such conditions such as headaches and muscle and joint pain. Blocking the inflammation can decrease the pain.

WHAT IS OVER-THE-COUNTER MEDICATION VS. PRESCRIPTION MEDICATION?

An over-the-counter (OTC) medication is one that is found in drugstores or supermarkets that you do not need a prescription for.

IS THERE REALLY A DIFFERENCE BETWEEN OVER-THE-COUNTER ANTI-INFLAMMATORY MEDICATIONS AND PRESCRIPTION ANTI-INFLAMMATORY MEDICATIONS?

There are a few differences. The first is the strength of each pill. For example, when you buy Advil, which is an OTC version of ibuprofen it comes in 200 mg pills. Prescription ibuprofen pills are 400 mg, 600 mg, or 800 mg. Other than that, there is no difference in the drug. Some NSAIDS are not over-the-counter because either the FDA (Food and Drug Administration) did not approve them or the company that makes them chose not to make an over-the-counter version.

WHAT ARE NSAID CREAMS OR OINTMENTS?

Some NSAIDS are sold in a cream or ointment form. These are not proven to have much effect. Some patients do say that it helps when used in the hands, knees, and feet.

WHAT ARE SOME OF THE PROBLEMS WITH NSAIDS?

The biggest problem with NSAIDS is that they can cause a person to experience pain in the stomach. This is probably because NSAIDS affect acid production in the stomach. NSAIDS also can thin the blood. Generally, they are safe, though.

DO ALL NSAIDS HAVE THE RISK OF UPSETTING THE STOMACH?

A few newer NSAIDS such as meloxicam (Mobic) and celacoxib (Celebrex) claim to have less stomach symptoms.

BESIDES NSAIDS, WHAT ARE THE MORE COMMON PAIN RELIEVERS FOR ARTHRITIS?

Acetaminophen (Tylenol), tramadol (Ultram), and narcotics. Tylenol is very effective and safe and is available without a prescription. Tramadol is a non-narcotic pain reliever but needs a prescription. Narcotics are drugs that are based on the powerful drug group called opiates. The common narcotics are morphine, meperidine (Demerol), hydromorphone (Dilaudid), oxycodone, hydrocodone, and codeine.

WHAT ARE SOME OF THE PROBLEMS WITH NARCOTIC PAIN RELIEVERS?

The biggest problem is that people can get addicted to narcotics. A street opiate is actually heroin, which is made from morphine. All opiates have risks of addiction and dependency. They also make people drowsy and can cause slow breathing (respiratory depression) that can cause death.

WHAT ARE SOME OF THE NUTRITIONAL SUPPLEMENTS THAT ARE BEING SOLD FOR ARTHRITIS?

In recent years there have been various plant-based chemicals and nutritional supplements that have been proposed for arthritis. These include glucosamine, chondroitin sulfate, SAM-E, MSM, boswelia, and others. While many people say they help with their bone and joint flexibility and pain, there have been no good scientific studies proving their value.

DO GLUCOSAMINE AND CHONDROITIN SULFATE ACTUALLY WORK?

When they do work, no one knows why. Companies try to say these chemicals are the building blocks of cartilage and nutritionally support the joint but that claim simply has not been proven.

IF THERE ARE NO SCIENTIFIC STUDIES PROVING THE VALUE OF THESE SUPPLEMENTS, THEN WHAT SHOULD I DO?

There are still many patients who seem to get quite a lot of improvement in motion and decrease in pain from some of these products so many doctors feel it is a reasonable thing for a person to do for a short period of time to see if it helps.

DOES PHYSICAL THERAPY WORK FOR ARTHRITIS OF THE HIP?

Most specialists in the field know that physical therapy is not very helpful specifically for hip arthritis pain. That does not mean that physical therapy can't be valuable to teach walking and strengthen some muscles. It may not cure or delay the need for medications or surgery when specifically talking about the hip.

WHAT KIND OF SURGERY EXISTS FOR HIP ARTHRITIS?

Hip replacement, hip resurfacing, and hip arthroscopy.

LABRUM TEARS

ARE LABRUM TEARS SERIOUS?

We are getting more of an appreciation of labrum tears in recent years as the quality of MRI's has increased. An MRI is a very sensitive test that allows doctors to see the acetabular labrum. Before MRI's it was difficult to make this diagnosis.

ARE ALL LABRUM TEARS PAINFUL?

Probably not. We really don't know which ones are painful and in fact it is not very common to need treatment for labrum tears.

IF A LABRUM TEAR IS THE CAUSE OF PAIN, WHAT IS THE TREATMENT?

Generally the first form of treatment is to rest the hip from activities that were causing the pain. The symptoms from a labrum tear frequently get better over time.

WHAT IF REST DOES NOT WORK?

Then surgery may be an option.

WHAT TYPE OF SURGERY IS THERE FOR A LABRUM TEAR?

Usually the surgery is arthroscopy of the hip. Arthroscopy of the hip is not as common as arthroscopy of the knee and is a more complex procedure. Not many Orthopaedic Surgeons do arthroscopy of the hip. When it is done, the surgeon trims the tear to a stable rim. That usually takes care of the pain. Sometimes the torn labrum can be reattached to the bone.

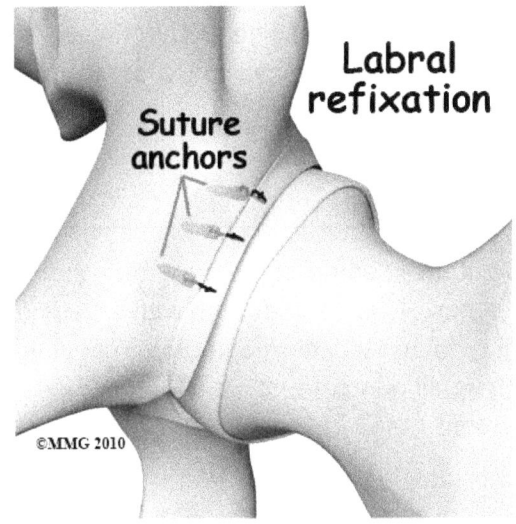

Labrum tears can be removed or repaired

HIP IMPINGEMENT (FEMOROACETABULAR IMPINGEMENT)

WHAT IS HIP IMPINGEMENT OR FEMOROACETABULAR IMPINGEMENT?

This problem is a relatively new diagnosis. It is a new way of looking at an early form of a specific type of arthritis. Some surgeons have proposed that this early type of arthritis can be treated with minimally invasive techniques that hopefully avoid a hip replacement. This problem is often referred to by the abbreviation FAI.

WHAT EXACTLY IS THE PROBLEM IN FAI?

The outer edge of the ball and socket joint is narrowed. This gives the appearance that the joint in this area is squeezed or impinged. It really isn't, though. It is just rubbing in a small area. Sometimes the cause of the narrowing is on the acetabular (socket side) and sometimes it is on the femoral (ball) side. Other times, extra bone forms on either the acetabulum or femur to cause an impingement or pinching of the joint.

WHAT IS THE TREATMENT OF FAI?

The treatment is to cut away some of the bone on either the acetabulum or the femur. This can be done with a traditional open operation with a full incision (called an osteotomy) or with hip arthroscopy through small puncture holes. Both methods are acceptable for treatment.

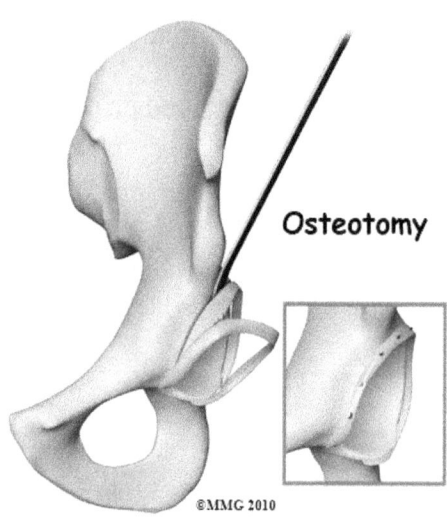

Some surgeons remove bone in FAI with an operation that requires a larger scar.

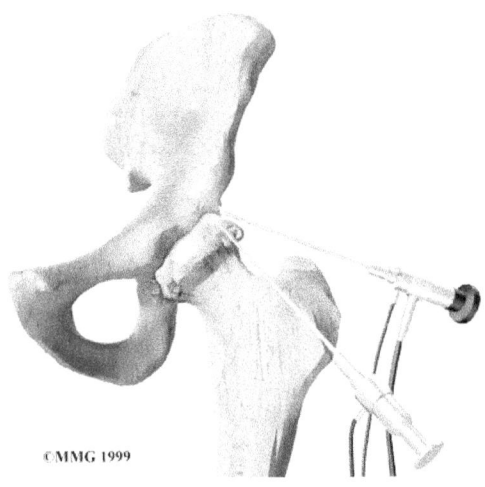

Some operations for FAI can be done arthroscopically with a smaller incision

WHY DON'T SURGEONS JUST DO HIP REPLACEMENT AS THE FIRST TREATMENT FOR FAI?

If cutting away the bone takes care of the pain, then you may avoid a hip replacement. Hip replacements are good to avoid or delay because even though new hip replacements last a long time, they do not last forever. Also, if the person can keep their own joint, there are more activities they can do than with a hip replacement.

DOES FAI EVENTUALLY GO ON TO MORE SEVERE HIP ARTHRITIS THAT WILL NEED HIP REPLACEMENT?

We really don't know the answer to this, but it probably does eventually.

AVASCULAR NECROSIS

HOW IS AVASCULAR NECROSIS TREATED?

Avascular necrosis of the femoral head is treated differently based on how early the diagnosis is made. To decide upon treatment, the surgeon "stages" the avascular necrosis. This means the person with avascular necrosis is placed into a severity category. There are 5 categories but in general you can think of it as two categories- early and late/advanced avascular necrosis.

HOW IS EARLY AVASCULAR NECROSIS TREATED?

In the early stages the surgeon tries to drill holes in the femoral head to bring blood into the dead area. This is called a "core decompression."

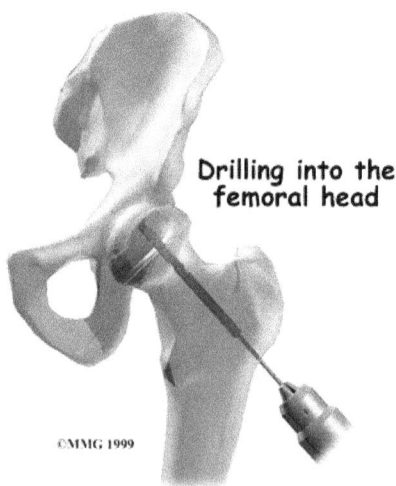

Drilling into the femoral head

Drilling holes in the bone in avascular necrosis may increase the blood supply and decrease pain

IS A CORE DECOMPRESSION A BIG OPERATION?

Of course, any operation of the hip can be considered big but as compared to a hip replacement, it is much smaller. A one-inch incision is made and some drill holes are put in the bone.

WHAT IS THE RECOVERY AFTER A CORE DECOMPRESSION?

The recovery tends to be quick- about 3-4 weeks. The problem is that the operation only works in a small number of patients. Therefore. after the recovery period, many patients are left with pain.

IF SO FEW PATIENTS DO WELL WITH A CORE DECOMPRESSION, THEN WHY IS IT DONE?

If you can do a small operation and avoid a hip replacement, then it is worth it.

IF HIP REPLACEMENTS ARE SO GOOD, WHY WOULD YOU WANT TO AVOID THEM IN AVASCULAR NECROSIS IN A YOUNG PATIENT?

Hip replacements are made of metal and plastic and ceramic. Eventually they wear out and the younger the patient, the more years they have to live, so the more years the hip replacement has to survive. Also, a hip replacement has a fair amount of blood loss and other potential complications that are more common than with a core decompression. In general, a core decompression is done to save the patient's own hip, because what you have is better than what we replace it with.

IF A CORE DECOMPRESSION DOES NOT RELIEVE THE PAIN IN THE HIP IN AVASCULAR NECROSIS, WHAT IS THE NEXT STEP?

A total hip replacement.

HOW IS LATE OR ADVANCED AVASCULAR NECROSIS TREATED?

Most people will treat late avascular necrosis with a hip replacement.

HIP INFECTIONS

WHAT ARE THE SYMPTOMS OF A HIP INFECTION?

Pain in the hip is often the first sign of a hip infection. Many patients do not get a fever so new pain, after a hip replacement has healed can be the only symptom. Sometimes there is hip or thigh swelling. Failure of the wound to heal early after the surgery can be a sign of infection.

HOW IS THE DIAGNOSIS OF A HIP INFECTION MADE?

Hip infections can be diagnosed or discovered by a history and physical exam with blood tests, x-ray type tests, or removing fluid from the joint.

WHAT BLOOD TESTS CAN HELP FIND OUT IF THERE IS A HIP INFECTION?

There are three common tests done. (1) a Complete Blood Count (CBC)- this tells whether there are white cells that increase in number in an infection. The problem with a CBC is that white cells can also increase in some non-infectious conditions. (2) C-Reactive Protein (CRP)- this is a very sensitive test that, if positive, almost always means there is an infection (3) ESR- this is also a sensitive test although not quite as good as a CRP. Most doctors get all three tests.

WHAT X-RAY TYPE TESTS CAN HELP FIND OUT IF THERE IS A HIP INFECTION?

In general, x-ray tests or imaging tests like a CT scan or an MRI don't give direct information about an infection. An x-ray only shows bone so that is not helpful unless in the rare case the infection is in the bone. An MRI can show a suggestion of infection by showing fluid collections.

HOW IS FLUID REMOVED FROM A HIP JOINT TO SEE IF THERE IS A HIP INFECTION?

Fluid from a hip is removed with a long needle. Most of the time this is done in a part of a hospital or medical building that has special x-rays to guide the doctor to make sure he or she is in the right place. Some doctors, based on experience, don't need this x-ray guidance.

WHAT IS AN INFECTION IN A "NATIVE" HIP?

A "native" hip infection is an infection in a hip that never had surgery before.

WHAT IS A PERIPROSTHETIC INFECTION?

This is an infection in a hip that had previous surgery where some type of metal was put in. The metal that is put in is called either an "implant" or a "prosthesis." Screws that fix hip fractures and hip replacements are both examples of implants/prostheses. The word "peri" means "around." Therefore a periprosthetic infection of the hip is an infection around an implant or prosthesis.

WHAT IS THE RECOMMENDED TREATMENT OF A NATIVE HIP INFECTION?

Most of the time a person will need an operation to open the hip joint and drain the infection out. Then antibiotics by intravenous (bloodstream) are given for a certain amount of time and then antibiotics by mouth are sometimes continued.

WHAT EVENTUALLY BECOMES OF A JOINT THAT GETS INFECTED?

It depends on how aggressive the bacteria are and how extensive the infection is. Most cases are cured with one operation and one course of antibiotics. Some patient do require multiple operations, though.

CAN YOU REPLACE A HIP IN A JOINT THAT WAS PREVIOUSLY INFECTED?

Generally, it is not recommended. There are situations when someone had an infection many decades earlier and now the infection is cured. Even those patients are probably at high risk and it may not be recommended to do a hip replacement. Each person, though, needs his or her own evaluation by a doctor. It is important to make sure there is no small area of infection remaining.

WHAT IS THE RECOMMENDED TREATMENT OF A HIP REPLACEMENT THAT BECOMES INFECTED?

Treatment of hip infections is very individualized. Sometimes antibiotics by mouth or intravenous are the only treatment. The next level would be to do another operation to wash the joint out with antibiotic fluid. The final level is to remove the infected hip replacement, put in a temporary spacer coated with antibiotics, and then put a new hip replacement after the infection clears. I can not emphasize enough how different the plan is based on the nature of the infection.

TREATMENT OF CHILDREN'S HIP PROBLEMS THAT LEAD TO PROBLEMS AS ADULTS

WHAT TYPE OF DOCTOR TREATS THESE CHILDREN'S HIP PROBLEMS?

Just as pediatricians are the doctors that treat children, there is a section of orthopaedics called pediatric orthopaedics that treats hip problems in children. General orthopaedic surgeons are well qualified to treat many of these conditions as well. It depends on the doctor's training and experience.

HOW IS DEVELOPMENTAL OR CONGENITAL DYSPLASIA OF THE HIP DDH/CDH) TREATED?

This is usually treated with different types of bracing. Sometimes, in difficult cases, surgery is needed.

WHAT TYPE OF SURGERY IS NEEDED SOMETIMES IN DDH/CDH?

The surgery is very complex and done by pediatric orthopaedic surgeons. Sometimes the bones of the pelvis and the femur need to be broken and fixed in different positions. It is not common to need this surgery, fortunately.

HOW IS LEGG-CALVÉ PERTHES TREATED?

It is treated with modification of activities (rest), traction (in bed with weights pulling on the leg), and sometimes braces to keep the hip in specific positions.

HOW IS SLIPPED CAPITAL FEMORAL EPIPHYSIS (SCFE) TREATED?

It is treated with surgery. The surgeon puts screws in the hip to prevent the bone from slipping anymore.

WHAT HAPPENS TO PATIENTS WITH CHILDHOOD HIP PROBLEMS WHEN THEY REACH ADULTHOOD?

The problem with these three hip problems is that many of the people who got them end up needing hip replacement at any time from their late 20's onward.

HIP FRACTURES (BROKEN HIP)

WHAT ACTUALLY BREAKS IN A HIP FRACTURE?

Of the two bones that make up the hip joint, it is the femur that breaks in a hip fracture. The femur starts in the hip joint and goes to the knee. When the upper part of the femur breaks, it is called a hip fracture.

WHY DOES A HIP ACTUALLY BREAK?

Most hip fractures happen because the bone got too thin because of a problem called osteoporosis. Of course, a fall from a tall height or a car accident can cause a hip to break.

WHAT IS OSTEOPOROSIS?

Osteoporosis is a problem with bone where it essentially thins out and gets weaker. For reasons related to changes in women, as they get older, they get more osteoporosis than men.

HOW ARE HIP FRACTURES TREATED?

Nearly all hip fractures are treated with surgery.

HOW IS THE TREATMENT CHOICE MADE IN HIP FRACTURES?

It depends on where in the hip the fracture is. Fractures get fixed with screws, plates, pins, rods, or with some type of hip replacement. For those readers who want more information- here it is. Fractures that are closer to the ball or head of the femur tend to get replaced. Fractures lower down tend to get fixed with screws, rods, plates or some type of hardware.

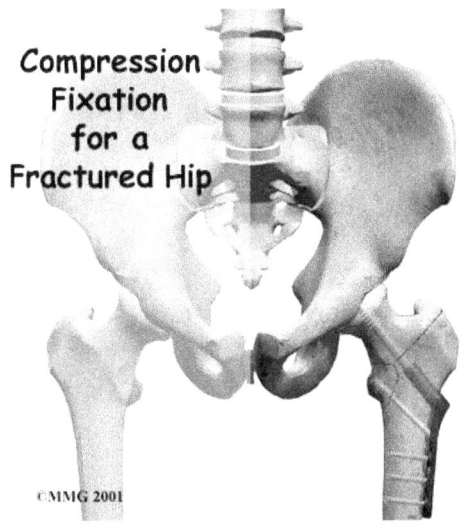

Compression Fixation for a Fractured Hip

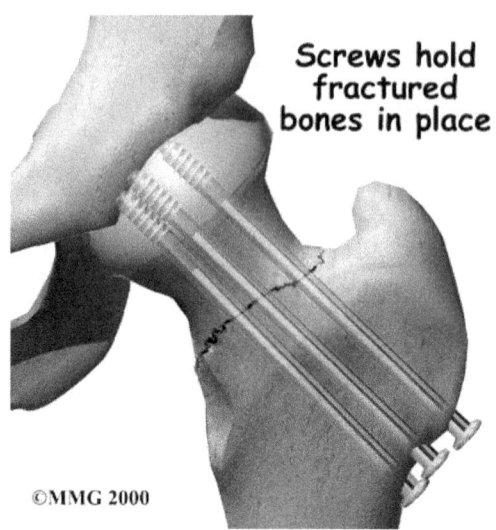

Different types of hip fractures require different types of operations

WHAT TYPE OF REPLACEMENT IS DONE FOR CERTAIN HIP FRACTURES?

When hip fractures need a replacement, there are two types of replacements. There is a partial replacement, also called a hemi-replacement. In fact the real medical name is a hemiarthroplasty. The word "arthro" means "joint" and the word "plasty" means to change or modify. The other replacement operation is a total hip replacement. Which one you get depends on many factors. If you have arthritis in the hip that was fractured then you will probably get a total hip replacement. Some surgeons feel that active patients do better with total hip replacements vs. hemiarthroplasties but both operations are recommended.

AFTER HIP FRACTURE SURGERY, WHAT CAN A PERSON EXPECT?

In general people are not very happy after an operation for a hip fracture whether it was fixed with screws or replacements. This is probably because the fracture causes a lot of muscle damage and it takes a long time to recover. There are many schools of thought concerning advice after a hip fracture. Some surgeons have you put all your weight on the leg and some don't. One thing for sure, expect a long recuperation period- as long as 6 months!

HIP TENDONITIS

WHAT IS HIP TENDONITIS?

Hip tendonitis is not a common problem. Sometimes tendons deep in the hip joint are strained from an injury that causes pain.

HOW IS HIP TENDONITIS TREATED?

Hip tendonitis is usually treated with rest and anti-inflammatory medications. Sometimes physical therapy helps.

DOES HIP TENDONITIS EVER NEED SURGERY?

No.

HIP BURSITIS

HOW IS HIP BURSITIS TREATED?

The first time you get bursitis you are usually treated with oral anti-inflammatory medications. It is very common for the doctor to inject the bursa with steroids. These injections can be very helpful.

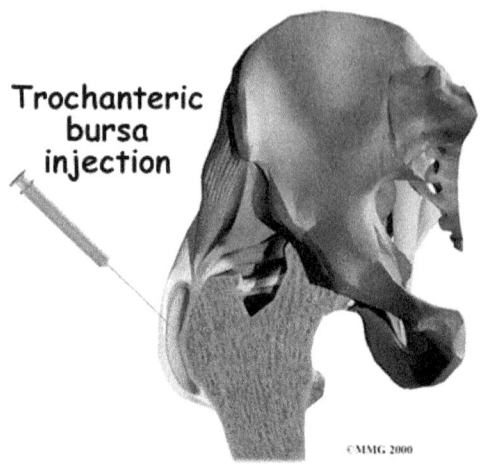

A hip bursa injection is easily done in the office

DOES HIP BURSITIS EVER NEED SURGERY?

Very rarely and almost never.

HIP REPLACEMENT SURGERY

WHAT IS A HIP REPLACEMENT?

A hip replacement is an operation where a surgeon opens your hip joint, removes part of the hip joint and puts in metal, plastic, or ceramic parts made by a company. It is also called a hip arthroplasty.

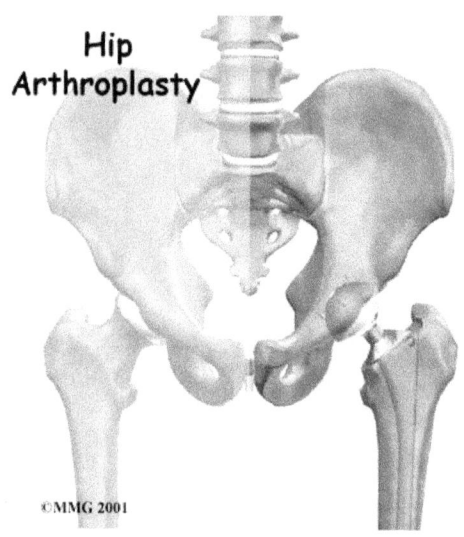

HOW LONG HAVE HIP REPLACEMENTS BEEN AROUND?

The modern history of joint replacement can be traced to the early 1960's. While there were some types of joint replacement before that time, it was not until a British surgeon, Sir John Charnley, worked out many of the issues and invented the current hip replacement. There have been improvements since that time but Charnley's basic design is still the best.

WHAT KIND OF DOCTOR DOES HIP REPLACEMENTS?

An orthopaedic surgeon does this surgery. This is a doctor who went to medical school and then did a minimum of five years of training in Orthopaedic Surgery called a "residency." Some surgeons, after their residency, do an extra year, of training called a fellowship in joint replacement. This extra year is a personal choice and is not required to be qualified to do joint replacements.

WHAT TYPE OF COMPANY MAKES A HIP REPLACEMENT?

The type of company that makes joint replacement is often called a "device manufacturer."

WHAT ARE SOME OF THE MORE POPULAR COMPANIES THAT MAKE HIP REPLACEMENTS?

In alphabetical order they are Biomet, Depuy/JNJ, DJO, Stryker, Wright Medical, and Zimmer

ARE THERE DIFFERENCES BETWEEN COMPANIES AND THEIR MODELS OF HIP REPLACEMENTS?

Each company will tell you there are many differences between their products and the other companies. The differences are mainly related to a surgeon's preference in how they feel the joint replacement should fix to the bone. From the point of view of results, though, they are remarkably similar in their success.

WHAT ARE ALL THE PARTS OR COMPONENTS OF A HIP REPLACEMENT?

There are four parts or components that go into a hip replacement. They are the cup (acetabular shell), the cup liner (acetabular insert), the stem (femoral stem), and the head (femoral head).

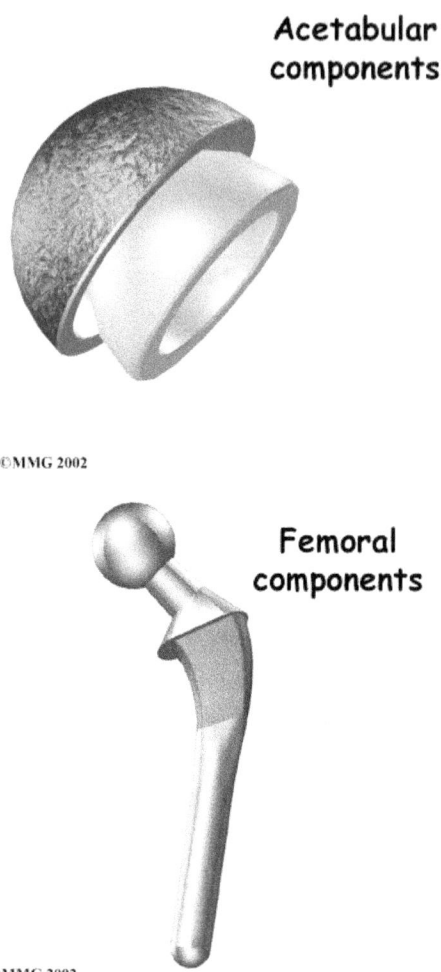

The acetabular components are the metal shell and liner. The femoral components are the femoral head and stem.

WHAT MATERIALS ARE A HIP REPLACEMENT MADE OF?

The acetabular shell is made of a metal, either titanium or a cobalt-chrome. The acetabular insert is made of either a plastic (called polyethylene), ceramic, or metal.

WHAT ARE THE MOST COMMON CONFIGURATIONS HIP REPLACEMENTS?

There are two most common configurations of hip replacements. These are (1) metal acetabular shell/polyethylene liner/metal femoral head/metal femoral stem and (2) metal acetabular shell/polyethylene liner/ceramic femoral head/metal stem.

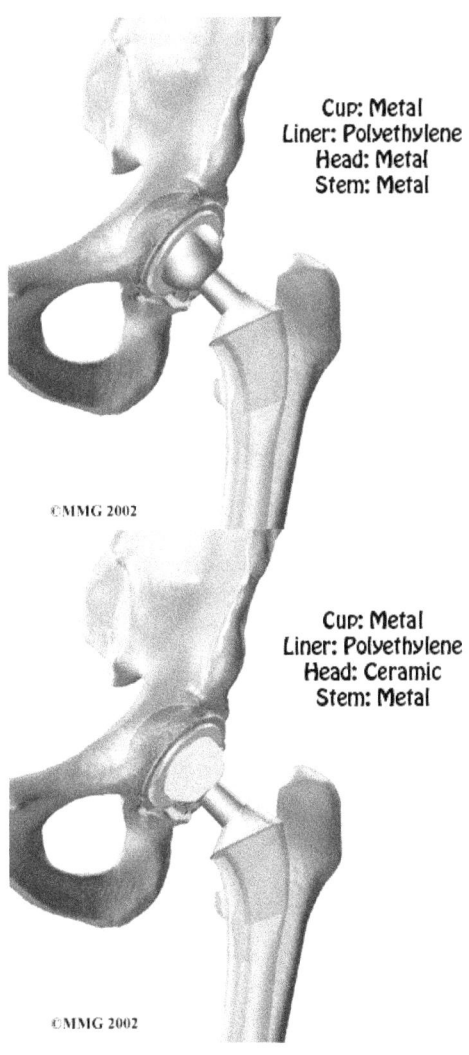

Cup: Metal
Liner: Polyethylene
Head: Metal
Stem: Metal

Cup: Metal
Liner: Polyethylene
Head: Ceramic
Stem: Metal

WHAT ARE OTHER HIP REPLACEMENT CONFIGURATIONS?

Metal shell/ceramic liner/ceramic femoral head/metal femoral stem

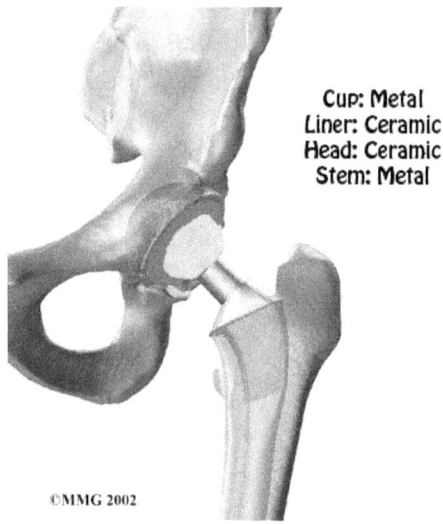

Cup: Metal
Liner: Ceramic
Head: Ceramic
Stem: Metal

Metal shell/metal acetabular liner/metal femoral head/metal femoral stem

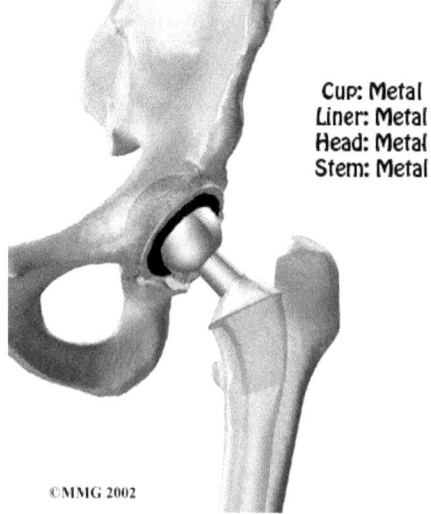

Cup: Metal
Liner: Metal
Head: Metal
Stem: Metal

THERE ARE SO MANY MIXES AND MATCHES HERE- HOW IS IT DECIDED WHAT I GET

Your surgeon will discuss your options and his or her preferences for you and why. If he/she doesn't then definitely bring this up as a discussion point.

CAN YOU SHOW ME THE DIFFERENCE OF EACH CONFIGURATIO?

The following reviews an understanding of the differences in safety and lifespan of the different configurations. Use this only as a discussion point with your surgeon.

Polyethylene liner/metal head: high safety/moderate lifespan/low cost/no complications

Polyethylene liner/ceramic head: high safety/high lifespan/high cost/no complications

Ceramic liner/ceramic head: high safety/high lifespan/highest cost/complications- 5% of the time make a squeaking sound when the patient walks

Metal liner/metal head: low safety/high lifespan/highest cost/complications-metal in blood and around the hip

IF METAL-ON-METAL IS NOT AS SAFE THEN WHY IS IT USED?

It is not used often. In general, it was originally used for all the right reasons. Metal-on-metal allows for large femoral heads that give better motion and lower dislocation rate. The complications of metal ions in the blood and metal deposits in the soft tissues around the hip were unexpected. Since some companies had no problems with metal-on-metal replacements. It is believed, at this time, that he metal-on-metal from certain specific companies is very safe.

HOW IS THE CUP PUT IN AND FIXED TO THE BONE?

The surgeon uses a tool called a reamer to core out the cup in a semicircle shape. The semicircle has a certain diameter and the shell is a tiny bit smaller in diameter. It is press fit into the cored out area. Sometimes the surgeon uses screws to reinforce the fixation.

HOW IS THE FEMORAL COMPONENT PUT IN AND FIXED TO THE BONE?

Most surgeons use a "cementless" technique. The surgeon uses tools called reamers and broaches to shape out the inside of the femur. The femoral stem is a bit smaller than the shape that was formed and is press fit into the femur. The bone then grows directly into the metal. In patients who have poor quality bone or for some other reason, the surgeon can "cement" a stem into the bone. The surgeon fills the canal with a doughy product similar to tile grout. The stem is placed into this cement. The cement then hardens. Cementless replacements tend to last longer than cemented ones.

DO ANY OF THE PARTS WEAR OUT?

The metal shell, femoral stem, and femoral head do not wear out. The polyethylene liner can wear out.

IF A POLYETHYLENE LINER CAN WEAR OUT, THEN WHY DON'T SURGEONS USE SUBSTITUTES FOR POLYETHYLENE?

There have been attempts at substituting the polyethylene. These have included ceramic liners and metal liner. The problems have been that ceramic liners with ceramic heads can cause a high number of squeaks when the patient walks. Metal liners with metal heads can cause metal ions in the bloodstream and metal to be deposited in the area around the hip.

CAN I REQUEST ONE TYPE OR ANOTHER OF CONFIGURATION?

You can. The surgeon should explain to you why he/she is choosing one type of hip for you vs. another. Keep in mind, you may want a certain configuration but the surgeon does not have to agree to put that into you. If you disagree with your surgeon, then seek another opinion. Be careful, though, because the first surgeon may be correct. Be wise in your research.

WHO MONITORS THE QUALITY OF THESE JOINT REPLACEMENTS?

The FDA.

WHAT IS THE FDA?

The FDA or Food and Drug Administration is a federal (national) government agency that monitors and approves the use and safety of food, drugs, and devices in many areas but especially in healthcare.

HOW DO I KNOW THE PRODUCT IS SAFE?

Device companies adhere to very strict safety guidelines set forth by the FDA. It is also common for these companies to seek the expert opinion of practicing surgeons to improve the products and assure their safety. The Orthopaedic device industry has a remarkable safety record over many decades.

CAN I BE ALLERGIC TO A HIP REPLACEMENT?

Allergies to metal do exist, but they are very rare. It is unlikely your hip will fail due to a metal allergy.

HOW IS METAL ALLERGY TESTED?

There are allergy specialists that test this with skin tests. Metal allergy is so rare that most surgeons don't recommend routine testing.

I HAVE HEARD ABOUT "RECALLS." WHAT ARE THESE ABOUT?

A very small number of hip replacements have either had some manufacturing problems or simply haven't worked well for unknown reasons. When this occurs, there is mandatory reporting to the FDA. Sometimes, if the FDA feels the issue is serious enough, it issues a "recall." A recall in the device industry is complex. It generally means that all hip products that have not been sold need to be returned to the company. Patients who have already received these are made aware of potential problems that could happen with the products they have. The specific instructions for patients depend on the problem and the findings of the FDA.

WHO REALLY CHOOSES MY JOINT REPLACEMENT?

Either your surgeon or the hospital the surgeon operates at decides on the hip replacement model. At most hospitals, it is a combination of both. A standard method is for the surgeons who do most of the hip replacements get together as a group and decide which model or models will be stocked in the hospital. They look at the success of the hip replacement, cost, safety, ease of use, and their own experiences with the various models.

HOW DO I KNOW IF I NEED A HIP REPLACEMENT?

Very few people actually "need" a hip replacement. You should look at it this way- Can you benefit from a hip replacement? If you have significant pain that is not relieved by medications or acceptable modifications in your activities then you should consider a hip replacement. There are many non-surgical options, such as modifying your activities, anti-inflammatory medications, use of a cane, pain medications, and sometime hip injections that can relieve your pain and increase your function.

HOW DO I "CARE" FOR A HIP REPLACEMENT TO MAKE IT LAST LONGER?

The main thing you can do to make a hip replacement last longer is to keep your weight low and limit activity that will cause the moveable surfaces to wear out.

WHAT KIND OF ACTIVITY SPECIFICALLY CAUSES A HIP REPLACEMENTTO WEAR OUT?

Running, jumping, too much walking, too much cycling.

IN GENERAL, IF I LOOK AT ACTIVITY IN THREE WAYS, LOW, MEDIUM, AND HIGH LEVELS, THEN HOW LONG CAN A HIP REPLACEMENT LAST?

Let's answer this in the following way. If a surgeon replaces 100 joints in the year 2000, at what year would the 25th one fail, leaving 75 still around? In low activity people, 25% of hip replacements will fail in 25 years, in medium activity people, 25% of hip replacements will fail in 18 years, and in high activity people, 25% of hip replacements will fail in 8-12 years. These are estimates but are pretty good.

WHAT IS THE AVERAGE AGE OF PEOPLE WHO GET HIP REPLACEMENTS?

This depends on the community. The average age does not really matter. Probably the most common age group is 70-80 but there are many people who need hip replacement younger and older than that.

IS SOMEONE TOO YOUNG TO GET A HIP REPLACEMENT?

The answer to that is no. If a young person, in their twenties has a bad hip and has absolutely intolerable pain restricting them to a wheelchair, then a hip replacement can be considered. We try our hardest, though, to delay hip replacements by using alternatives for as long as possible.

IS SOMEONE TOO OLD TO GET A HIP REPLACEMENT?

The answer is no. If a 90 year old person has intolerable pain from hip problems and is healthy, then a hip replacement can be considered,

IS SOMEONE TOO "SICK" TO GET A HIP REPLACEMENT?

Yes. At any age, if a person's medical problems make them at a high serious risk of death or other complications then, except is very specific situations, hip replacement surgery may not be offered.

IS A HIP REPLACEMENT A "DANGEROUS" OPERATION?

Comparing it to other major operations, hip replacement surgery is not dangerous. It is done in a controlled setting by a special team. By dangerous, I am referring to the risk of a patient dying or getting a serious life-changing injury. That is not common in hip replacement.

HOW LONG IS THE SURGERY?

Depending upon the surgeon, a hip replacement takes between one to two and a half hours.

ARE THERE DIFFERENT SURGICAL METHODS OF REPLACING A HIP?

Yes. In addition to which company's hip replacement model is chosen, there are different surgical approaches to the hip. The most common approaches are posterior, direct anterior, and anterior-lateral. A surgical approach is the specific method used to replacement the hip.

WHAT ARE THE DIFFERENCES BETWEEN THESE SURGICAL APPROACHES?

The posterior approach enters the hip from the back of the hip, the direct anterior enters from the front, and the anterior-lateral enters initially from the side and then the front.

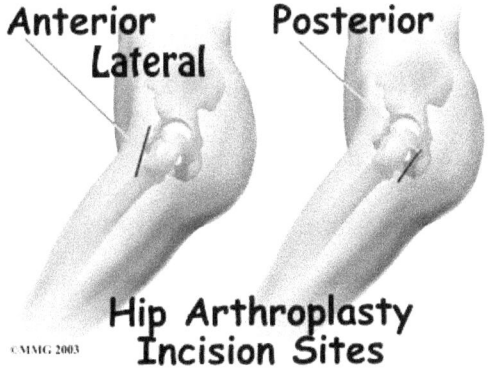

WHICH APPROACH SHOULD I CHOOSE?

You shouldn't. You should choose the surgeon. In expert hands, 3-6 months after surgery there is absolutely no difference in the results from these approaches. Since you are trying to get a successful result for over two decades some subtle differences between the approaches should not sway your decision. The direct anterior and posterior approaches tend to have early recovery time by a few weeks but slightly higher complications than the anterior-lateral such as getting dislocations and leg lengths. Keep in mind-in expert hands there is really no difference at all between the three approaches in recovery and complications.

CAN ROBOTS DO THIS SURGERY?

Not really at this time. There are some early robotic assistants that are being developed to assist in the placement of the hip replacements but whether or not this technology catches on is not clear yet. The problem is that in good surgical hands, assuming there is no infection; hip replacement surgery is 98% successful. The robot would have to improve on that in some way.

WHAT ARE THE SURGICAL STEPS IN A HIP REPLACEMENT?

After the patient is placed on the operating room table in the proper position, here are the steps:

- The skin is cleansed with a sterile solution
- The skin is cut with a scalpel (an incision)
- The muscles are separated or partially cut
- The hip joint popped out (dislocated)
- The femoral head is cut off

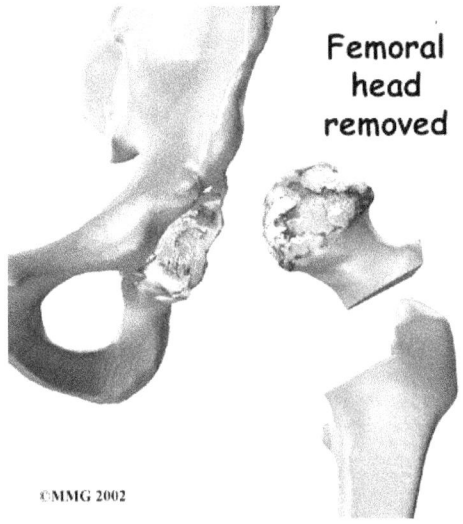

- The acetabulum is cleaned out (reamed)

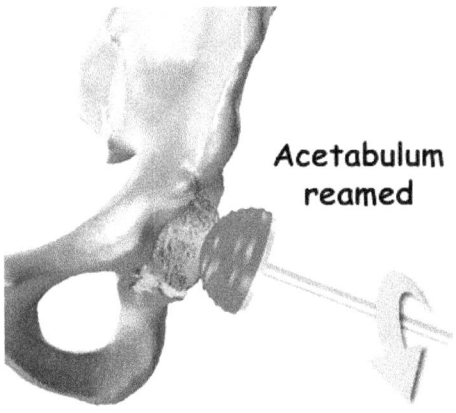

- The cup is inserted
- The liner is inserted

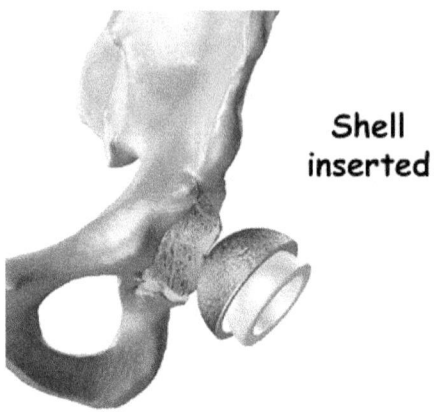

- The femoral stem is prepared (reamed and broached)

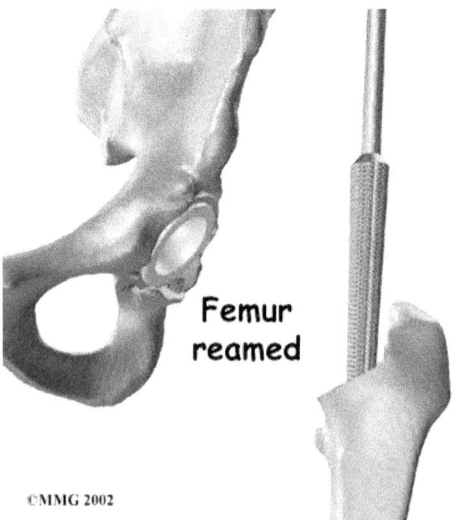

- The femoral stem is inserted

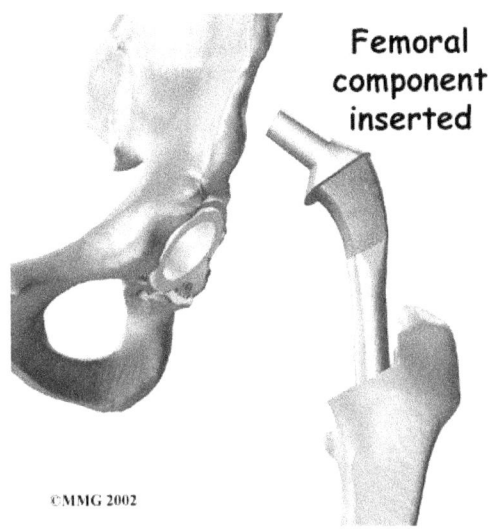

- The femoral head is inserted

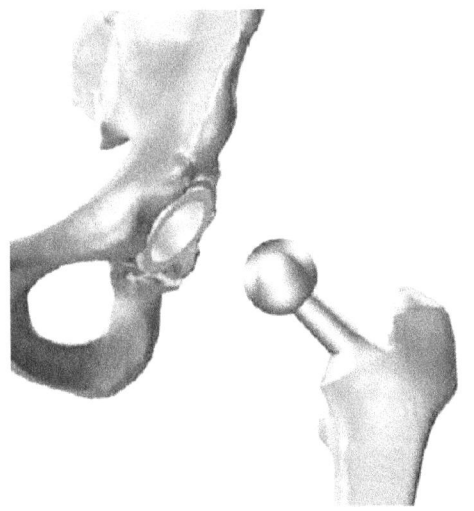

- The hip is popped back in (reduced)

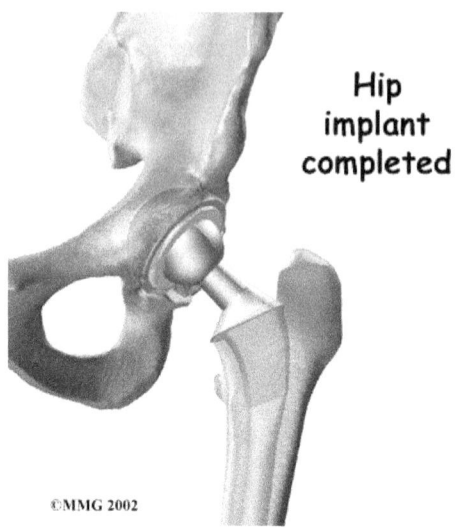

Hip implant completed

- The muscle and skin are closed and a dressing is applied.

WHAT ARE SOME OF THE COMPLICATIONS?

The major complications of hip replacements are dislocations, leg lengths, fractures, loosening, and infections.

WHAT IS A HIP DISLOCATION AFTER HIP REPLACEMENT?

A hip dislocation is when the ball pops out of the socket. This is immediately very painful and the person usually falls immediately. You would need to be transported to a hospital to treat this. The treatment is to go under anesthesia and have it popped back in. Sometimes surgery is needed to put in back it. When a person dislocates multiple times they sometimes need surgery to correct the reason it dislocates.

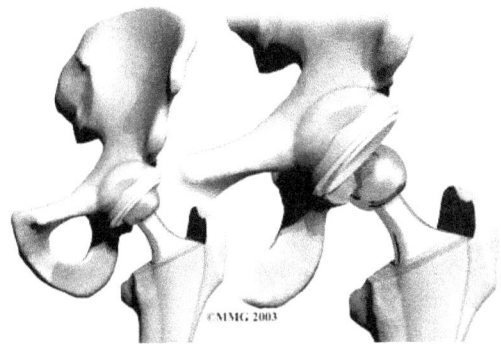

A hip dislocation after a hip replacement is very painful and often needs to be treated under anesthesia. The surgeon can pop it back in. Sometimes an operation is needed.

WHY DOES A HIP DISLOCATION HAPPEN AND HOW IS IT PREVENTED?

Hip dislocations can happen for a variety of reasons. The first reason is if the cup or stem is not placed in proper position. The second is the tightness or looseness that is in the hip. A loose joint can occur because the person is naturally loose or the surgeon put the hip in with loose tension. A third reason that a hip dislocates is that the patient who has the hip replacement puts the hip into positions that they were advised not to do causing it to pop op. The fourth reason is when the plastic of the cup wears out and causes the hip to dislocate.

HOW DOES A LEG LENGTH PROBLEM HAPPEN?

Most leg length problems after surgery cannot be avoided. We are trying to replace a natural hip with a man-made hip and sometimes it is not possible to correct everything. A hip is longer because the surgeon needed to lengthen the hip to make the muscles and ligaments tighter to give more stability to prevent a dislocation.

HOW AND WHEN DOES A FRACTURE (BROKEN BONE) OCCUR IN A HIP REPLACEMENT?

A fracture around a hip replacement can occur in the operating room or any time after surgery. In the operating room it can happen when a surgeon is preparing the thigh bone (femur) for the stem. The stem is usually press-fit into the bone and the tighter the fit, the more stable it is in the bone. If the bone quality is not great or the fit too tight then a fracture can occur. During the case the surgeon can fix the fracture, move on, and successfully complete the case. If a fracture happens after the surgery, it is usually from a fall. In that case a second operation to fix the bone or to take out the joint replacement and insert one that replaces the joint and fixes the fracture is used.

HOW DOES A HIP REPLACEMENT LOOSEN FROM ITS ATTACHMENT TO THE BONE?

Some loosen from infection. An infection separates the metal from the bone. Sometimes it loosens because wear and tear particles from the material, over time, separate the metal from the bone.

WHY DOES A HIP REPLACEMENT GET INFECTED?

No one really knows for sure. Sometimes an infection happens during the case despite very strict sterile environment. It also can happen in people who have sicknesses that make it more difficult for them to fight infection. These include diabetes, hepatitis, and HIV/AIDS. Other times, if you have an infection elsewhere in your body, that infection can travel to the replaced hip. Common origins of infections that can travel to the hip are skin, urine, lung, and blood infections.

HOW IS A TOTAL HIP REPLACEMENT INFECTION DIAGNOSED?

If an infection occurs within the first few weeks of surgery, sometimes the wound does not heal and fluid drains from the skin. This is often a sign of an infection. Once the hip heals and infection happens later, then it is more difficult to diagnose. Usually the surgeon starts by drawing blood tests discussed earlier like a white cell count (WBC), c-reactive protein (CRP), and erythrocyte sedimentation rate (ESR). Fluid is sometimes removed from the hip joint and sent to the lab to see if it contains bacteria. Sometimes special radiology tests such as a bone scan and white cell scan can help make the diagnosis.

WHAT IS THE TREATMENT OF AN INFECTED HIP REPLACEMENT?

It depends on how soon after the hip replacement was done that the hip got infected. It also depends on how long the infection was there. A combination of antibiotics and operations can be used to treat hip infections. Sometimes an operation to open the hip and clean out the joint, followed by antibiotics can cure the infection. In more difficult cases the surgeon may have to remove the original hip replacement, put in a temporary hip replacement coated with antibiotics, and then reinsert a new hip replacement after antibiotics are given for a period of time.

HOW FAST DOES IT TAKE TO RECOVER FROM A HIP REPLACEMENT?

It depends on your definition of the word "recover." I like to think of recovery from hip replacement surgery in three phases. The first is healing the wound and getting over the somewhat traumatic experience of surgery. This takes about 2 weeks. The next phase is early recovery. This is where you start to walk more, get more independent and in general begin to say to yourself that you are glad you had the surgery. You can get out of bed, walk around your house and community, get in and out of a car, and do similar things. This takes 2-6 weeks. The final phase is when you start doing so well where you forget you had a hip replacement and that takes about 3-6 months.

HOW QUICKLY CAN I GET UP OUT OF BED AND WALK AFTER SURGERY?

We now try to get the person up out of bed the first day. By the third day, after surgery you can possibly walk about 100 feet with a walker or crutches.

CAN I GO HOME AFTER THE SURGERY?

Most surgeons have rapid recovery programs with physical therapy working to make you independent to get out of bed, walk, and go home by the third to fifth day. This depends upon your total body health, upper body strength, and the safety of your home environment.

IF I DON'T GO HOME AFTER THE SURGERY, THEN WHERE DO I GO?

If you don't go home you will go to a rehabilitation facility. Other names for this are a nursing home, short-term care facility, extended care facility, or rehab home.

HOW DO I BENEFIT FROM PHYSICAL THERAPY?

Physical therapy is helpful to teach safe transferring out of bed, how to use the bathroom, teach precautions of how to place the hip, and retrain you how to walk normally again.

HOW BAD IS THE PAIN AFTER THE SURGERY?

It is very bad for 2-3 days. Let's call that on a scale of 1-10, where 1 is low pain and 10 is the highest pain, the pain after surgery is 8-10 for the first 3 days, 4-7 for up to two weeks, and 1-3 from 3-6 weeks. This is just a general guideline.

HOW IS THE PAIN RELIEVED AFTER SURGERY?

Usually, the pain is relieved by a variety of methods. Some surgeons give injections of pain medicines directly into the hip joint before the surgery ends. Then, surgeons will give one or more of the following- an intravenous pain pump that is controlled by the patient, pain medication injections orpain medicines by mouth. Surgeons work hard to find the right mix of controlling your pain but not giving you too much pain medicine that can make you too tired or can interfere with your breathing.

ASIDE FROM PAIN MANAGEMENT, WHAT OTHER TYPES OF TREATMENTS ARE GIVEN TO ME AFTER SURGERY?

The surgeon does three important things after the surgery. With your medical doctor, he/she restarts many of your medications for your general medical problems like high blood pressure and diabetes, monitor your blood pressure and laboratories to see if you need a blood transfusion, and thin your blood to prevent blood clots that can develop after hip replacement surgery.

WHY IS MY BLOOD THINNED?

Developing blood clots in the legs is a common complication of hip replacement. Doctors will either give you medications or use leg compression devices to prevent this. This is important because a blood clot in the legs can travel to the lungs and cause problems breathing or even death.

HOW DO I CHOOSE A SURGEON AND WHAT ARE HIS/HER QUALIFICATIONS TO DO A HIP REPLACEMENT?

There are many ways people choose surgeons. A medical or family doctor can make a recommendation and so can a friend who either had surgery or knows someone who did. However you get to the surgeon, you will still have to make your own decision. Ask yourself these questions:

DO YOU LIKE THE SURGEON' GENERAL APPROACH?

This is a very important part of your interview process. You need to connect to medical people who take care of you. Is the surgeon thoughtful and caring? Is he/she attentive to you. Are you pleased with his/her explanations to your questions?

DID HE/SHE TAKE A THOROUGH HISTORY AND DO A COMPLETE EXAMINATION?

A quick discussion, simple exam, and then the statement "you need surgery" is probably not what you are looking for in a surgeon. A careful history where the surgeon makes sure he/she is aware of all your past and current complaints and medical problems is a good sign that you will be well taken care of. This goes the same for a physical exam that is complete. Good surgeons all start this way.

DID YOU LIKE THE WAY HE/SHE EXPLAINED ALL THE STEPS?

If he/she cannot explain the surgery well, then there are two reasons for this- either he/she does not know enough or does not care enough to talk to you. Both are important when you choose a surgeon. He/she needs to be knowledgeable and needs to impart that knowledge to you.

DO YOU KNOW WHERE THE SURGEON TRAINED?

Where the surgeon trained can be helpful but you as the patient do not always know where in the country are the best places for training in hip replacement surgery. The best way is for you to find out where your surgeon trained and go on the Internet and research that place. It will be clear whether it is a top training location.

DID HE/SHE DO SOME TYPE OF JOINT REPLACEMENT FELLOWSHIP?

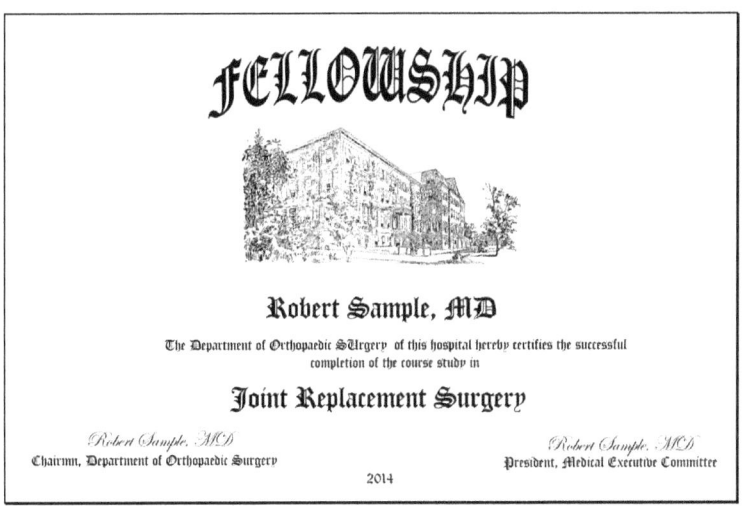

Look for a diploma in the office

While not a requirement, people who did a joint replacement fellowship after the general orthopaedic training at least show an interest in specializing in joint replacement and a focus on joint replacement. It is definitely a plus to have a surgeon who obtained some type of advanced training.

DOES HE/SHE DO MORE THAN 25 HIP REPLACEMENTS A YEAR?

This is one of the most important questions. Surgeons who do a minimum of 25 joints replacements a year have better results and fewer complications than those who do less than that.

IS HE/SHE BOARD CERTIFIED BY THE AMERICAN BOARD OF ORTHOPAEDIC SURGEONS (ABOS)?

The American Board of Orthopaedic Surgeons (ABOS) is the only official organization that certifies Orthopaedic Surgeons. There are some imitation boards but the ABOS is the real thing. http://www.abos.org.

IS HE/SHE A MEMBER OF THE AMERICAN ACADEMY OF ORTHOPAEDIC SURGEONS?

The American Academy of Orthopaedic surgeons is a professional organization of orthopaedic surgeons in the United States. Membership requires board certification specifically with the American Board of Orthopaedic Surgeons. http://www.aaos.org.

IS HE/SHE A MEMBER OF THE AMERICAN ASSOCIATION OF HIP AND KNEE SURGEONS (AAHKS)?

Many orthopaedic surgeons who do a certain minimum number of joint replacements per year and display certain other qualifications belong to the American Association of Hip and Knee Surgeons (AAHKS). This is a positive to be a member but not a negative if he/she is not. http://www.aahks.org.

IS THE HOSPITAL A RESPECTED CENTER?

This can also be helpful. Many smaller, lesser-known hospitals actually have superb "Centers of Excellence" in joint replacement so you need to do your homework on the hospital as well.

DOES THE SURGEON HAVE ANY PUBLICATIONS IN THE FIELD?

Publications such as articles or books don't tell you anything about surgical skill but do give you an idea of the level of involvement your surgeon has in the specialty as a whole. This is a positive if they have publications but not a negative if they don't.

DOES HER/SHE LECTURE AT MEETINGS?

Many quality surgeons are asked to lecture at local, regional, and national meetings. This is a good sign.

WHO PAYS FOR ALL THE COSTS OF JOINT REPLACEMENT SURGERY?

Most of the time patients have health insurance. Keep in mind that there are many costs involved in a joint replacement. These include the hospital, surgeon, anesthesiologist, laboratory, pathologist, physical therapist, medical consultants, and possibly a rehabilitation center.

WHO ACTUALLY PAYS FOR THE JOINT REPLACEMENT MODEL ITSELF?

In the United States most hospital bills include the joint replacement product as part of the bill. Hospital bills are paid one of two ways. They are either paid as a single fee with everything included or a itemized way with every item adding to the cost. Many insurers such as Medicare, Medicaid, and managed care companies usually have relationships with hospitals were they pay a flat fee that includes everything related to the hip replacement including the operating room costs, joint replacement model, and all treatment in the hospital. These insurers pay the surgeon separately.

HOW MUCH DOES THE HOSPITAL AND THE DOCTOR ACTUALLY GET PAID?

Medicare and Medicaid tend to pay a hospital $12,000 to $18,000 for a hip replacement. Managed care companies can pay more or less than that depending on the contract they have with the hospital. The actual cost of the hip replacement model to the hospital is $3,000 to $8,000. That cost is subtracted from what the hospital gets from the insurance company. Certain private insurers can pay a hospital more than Medicare and Medicaid. The surgeon usually makes between $1,200 (Medicare) and $6,000 (private insurance). There, of course, are variations in this fee.

WHAT ARE ALL THE OTHER PARTS OF THE SURGERY THAT COST MONEY?

The anesthesiologist fee, medical consultants before, during, and after the hospital stay, rehabilitation facility costs, home care costs, and equipment such as a walker, crutches, cane, and bathroom and daily living accessories (reacher, raised toilet seat).

ARE THERE ANY PRECAUTIONS AFTER SURGERY THAT I NEED TO WORRY ABOUT?

Yes. After the surgery the surgeon and/or the physical therapist will review leg positions that you need to avoid. These positions depend on the specific approach used in your surgery but generally the precautions are not to move the hip excessively in certain positions. The positions you should avoid are best discussed with your specific surgeon. Bending the hip too much or rotating too much inward or outward are general precautions.

WHAT ABOUT ANTIBIOTICS FOR DENTAL WORK AND OTHER PROCEDURES?

For up to a year after surgery, it is generally recommended that you take antibiotics during the time you are having dental work or other invasive procedures.

WILL I TRIGGER METAL DETECTORS?

Probably. Your surgeon will give you a card alerting others that you have a hip replacement, but expect a pat down because anyone can make these kinds of cards.

HOW LONG IS THE HOSPITAL STAY?

The hospital stay is between 2-5 days. Then, you either go home or to a rehabilitation facility.

HOW DO I DECIDE TO GO TO A REHABILITATION FACILITY OR TO HOME?

Patients who are generally healthy, have good upper strength to allow them to go from sitting to standing easily, and have people living at home that can help them, can often go home. If you need more assistance with mobility and other daily activities, you may choose to go to a rehabilitation facility.

DO I GET PHYSICAL THERAPY AFTER I GET HOME?

Most people get what is called "home care services" after a hip replacement. A nurse who visits the home usually coordinates this. This is called a "homecare nurse." The services that the nurse coordinates are often physical therapy, occupational therapy, medical monitoring, and equipment.

WHAT IS THE DIFFERENCE BETWEEN PHYSICAL THERAPY AND OCCUPATIONAL THERAPY?

When working with hip replacement patients, physical therapy concentrates on leg strengthening, walking, safety going from a bed or chair to standing, and stairs. Occupational therapy concentrates on activities such as functioning in the kitchen and toilet, as well as dressing. These are often called "activities of daily living."

WHAT TYPE OF MEDICAL MONITORING HAPPENS AT HOME AFTER SURGERY?

The homecare nurse takes your blood pressure and evaluates your pulse and breathing. Also he/she evaluates the wounds for healing and infection as well as your legs for blood clots. Sometime he/she makes sure labs are done. All this is reported to your surgeon and/or medical doctor.

WHAT KIND OF EQUIPMENT DO I HAVE THE OPTION OF HAVING AT HOME?

Equipment after hip replacement is often called "durable medical equipment (DME)." The only important equipment is some type of device that assists in walking and in sitting on the toilet. Patients usually use a walker or crutches after the surgery. The crutches are either underarm crutches or forearm crutches (often called Lofstrand crutches). In the toilet you need to raise the height of the toilet seat because it is generally recommended not to sit too low when the hip will bend past a recommended amount. To do this you can get a simple raised toilet seat or what is called a 3-in-1 commode. Usually someone at the hospital arranges for you to get this equipment either before the surgery or after the surgery. Other types of equipment include a reacher to grasp objects, a device to help put your socks on, and a chair for the bath or shower. Some patients decide to install a bar in their bath or shower for safety.

WHAT ACTIVITIES CAN I DO AFTER A HIP REPLACEMENT?

Generally you can return to most of the activities you did before the hip replacement. This incudes walking, driving, golf, tennis, handball, light basketball, skiing, and more. You need to be aware that the more aggressive your activity is, the faster the hip will wear out. Also, return to any activities should proceed slowly and carefully.

WHAT ACTIVITIES SHOULD I STAY AWAY FROM AFTER A HIP REPLACEMENT?

You need to stay away from activities that can put your hip into positions that can (1) cause dislocations, (2) are too aggressive so that the hip can wear out early (such as jogging and running, and (3) extreme activities that can risk a fracture, such as high speed skiing or snowboarding.

WHEN CAN I DRIVE AFTER A HIP REPLACEMENT?

It depends on whether it's your right hip or your hip. It may be possible for you to drive as early as four weeks if it's your left and 6 weeks if its your right. Keep in mind that driving is a public activity where you put others at risk if you are not healthy enough to drive. I recommend practicing in an empty parking lot to evaluate this.

WHEN CAN I HAVE SEX AFTER A HIP REPLACEMENT?

You will probably be fairly tired after the surgery and you need to be aware of that. There are specific positions you need to avoid such as bending or rotating past a certain amount.

WHAT IS REVISION HIP SURGERY?

Hip revision surgery is when a hip replacement needs to be removed and a new one inserted.

WHEN IS HIP REVISION SURGERY NECESSARY?

If a hip replacement fails from infections, wearing out, or multiple dislocations then revision surgery is needed.

HOW SUCCESSFUL IS HIP SURGERY A SECOND OR THIRD TIME?

As a general rule, hip revision surgery is not as successful as first time or primary hip replacement surgery. Surgeons sometimes say that a patient goes down a level of function overall after a revision operation. This is hard to specifically define, but if you look at overall function from 1-5 with a successful primary hip replacement giving you a level of function of 5 then you will drop to a 4.

DO I NEED TO SEE A MEDICAL DOCTOR BEFORE THE SURGERY?

Yes. Medical problems need to be under control as much as possible before hip replacement. This is called "optimizing" your medical problems. The most common medical conditions that need to be optimized include diabetes, heart, lung, and vascular leg issues.

WHAT IS AN ANESTHESIOLOGIST?

An anesthesiologist is a doctor who specializes in giving you anesthesia and keeping you healthy during the surgery and in the recovery room (often called the Post-Anesthesia Unit or PACU).

WHAT KIND OF ANESTHESIA DO I GET FOR HIP REPLACEMENT SURGERY?

The anesthesiologist will offer you one of or a combination of three types of anesthesia: general, spinal, and regional.

WHAT IS GENERAL ANESTHESIA?

General anesthesia is when you are put to sleep and a machine breathes for you. It is very safe. There is a slightly increased risk of developing a fever originating in your lungs and even getting pneumonia.

WHAT IS SPINAL ANESTHESIA?

Spinal anesthesia is when the anesthesiologist puts a needle in your spine and injects numbing medicine to numb the lower part of your body. It has the advantage of giving you a slightly decreased risk of developing blood clots after surgery. Also when you wake up from general anesthesia you feel the surgery pain immediately. With spinal anesthesia the pain comes on gradually over hours after the surgery, allowing you to catch up to the pain with pain medications.

WHAT IS REGIONAL ANESTHESIA?

Regional anesthesia is numbing medicine injected into the leg directly. Hip replacement surgery is usually not done with regional anesthesia alone. Regional anesthesia is sometime used in addition to general anesthesia to help the patient with pain after he/she wakes up.

CAN YOU GIVE ME A SUMMARY OF WHAT HAPPENS, HOUR-BY-HOUR AND DAY-BY-DAY AFTER THE SURGERY?

After the surgery you are in the recovery room. There, the doctors and nurses will examine you very frequently to make sure you are healthy. Labs may be drawn and x-rays taken. When you are medically stable you will leave the recovery room to go to your floor. The first night will be difficult but with pain management medications you will be OK. The first day after surgery you will get blood drawn and physical therapy once or twice that day. The doctors and nurses will ask you to breath into a breathing exercise device (incentive spirometer) that inflates your lungs to avoid fever and pneumonia. Most hospitals use special leg pumps to prevent blood clots. The physical therapist will see you and start teaching you how to get out of bed. Over the next few days more of the same will happen. The doctors and nurses will make sure your wound is healing and all your labs are normal. The physical therapist will increase your activities. You will go home or to a rehabilitation facility when you are medically stable and can get out of bed safely, get to the bathroom, and walk around.

WILL I NEED A TRANSFUSION AFTER A HIP REPLACEMENT?

Some people do need a blood transfusion after a hip replacement. This depends usually on your blood count before surgery and your tendency to bleed. Some hospital have programs where you can donate your own blood prior to the surgery.

WHAT ARE THE SIGNS THAT A HIP REPLACEMENT IS STARTING TO FAIL?

Pain is usually the first sign of a hip replacement that fails. Sometimes limping is an early sign.

WHEN ARE THE STITCHES OR STAPLES REMOVED AFTER SURGERY?

Most surgeons have the stitches or staples removed at about two weeks.

HOW OFTEN WILL I SEE MY DOCTOR AFTER SURGERY?

Each surgeon has their own guidelines, but a common schedule is 2 weeks, 6 weeks, 3 months, one year, 2 years, and then 5 years, 10 years and so on.

SURFACE REPLACEMENTS, HIP ARTHROSCOPY, LABRUM TEARS, AND FEMOROACETABULAR IMPINGEMENT

WHAT IS A SURFACE REPLACEMENT?

A surface replacement is an operation that replaces the cup and only puts a cap on the femoral head? It does this with a metal cup and a metal head.

HOW LONG HAVE SURFACE REPLACEMENTS BEEN AROUND?

It is not a new operation. There have be a variety of surface replacements done since the 1950's.

WHY WOULD SOME SURGEONS RECOMMEND A SURFACE REPLACEMENT?

Most surgeons do not choose a surface replacement over a hip replacement for their patients. Those surgeons that choose a surface replacements say the advantages are that in a surface replacement you leave the patient's neck whereas in a hip replacement, the neck and head get replaced. By keeping the neck and the patient's normal anatomy the theory is that you have more of a chance to return to more normal walking and activity function. Also, there is another theory that the very large femoral heads in surface replacements may give the patient better function. Total hip replacements now offer similar large size femoral heads, though.

IS A HIP RESURFACING LESS INVASIVE THAN A TOTAL HIP REPLACEMENT?

Not really. The incision and the cutting of muscles and other tissues is about the same in both operations. Less bone is removed in a surface replacement but the difference is very small. Essentially these operations have the same level of invasiveness.

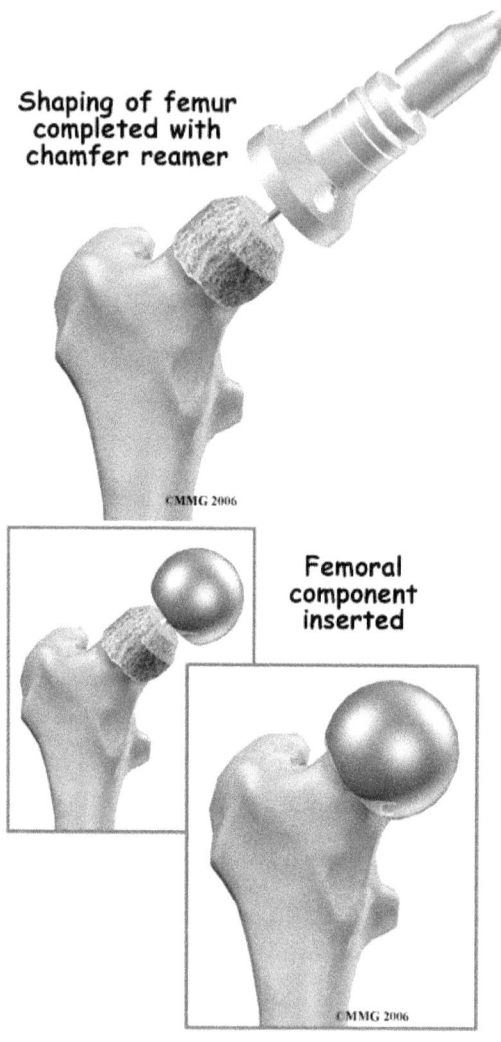

The steps to complete a surface replacement

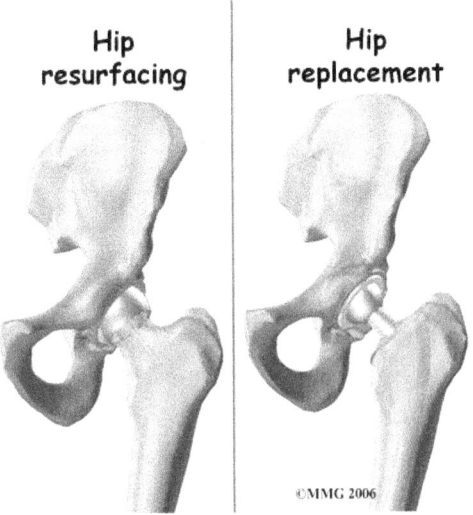

Hip resurfacing and replacement

IS THERE ANY SPECIFIC REASON NOT TO HAVE A HIP RESURFACING?

Yes. Since a resurfacing has a metal cup and a metal head it has the same potential complication of any metal-on-metal replacements, which are metal in the blood and in the soft tissues around the hip. This potential complication may be enough to decide not to have a surface replacement. Also, the reported long-term success results of total hip replacements are much longer than surface replacements.

WHEN WOULD SOMEONE RECOMMEND A SURFACE REPLACEMENT INSTEAD OF A HIP REPLACEMENT?

Certain young and active patients, according to some surgeons can benefit form the theoretical increased function a surface replacement can give. A vast majority of surgeons recommend a total hip replacement due to its excellent functional and safety results for so many decades.

WHAT IS HIP ARTHROSCOPY?

Hip arthroscopy is an operation where the surgeon puts 2-3 small puncture holes around the hip joint and place a device called an arthroscope in the hip joint. An arthroscope is a camera that takes pictures and video. The surgeon looks throughout the hip joint and if he/she sees a problem that can be fixed with tools inserted in other puncture holes. In comparison to knee arthroscopy, hip arthroscopy is not common. There are probably two reasons. The first is that there is little guarantee that these problems- labrum tear, femoroacetabular impingement, and loose bodies can be cured through a hip arthroscopy, while cartilage tears in the knees almost invariably get treated well with knee arthroscopy. We are just beginning to get an understanding of which disorders can be treated with hip arthroscopy. The second reason is that hip arthroscopy is not common and is technically difficult to do. Few surgeons are technically proficient at this procedure.

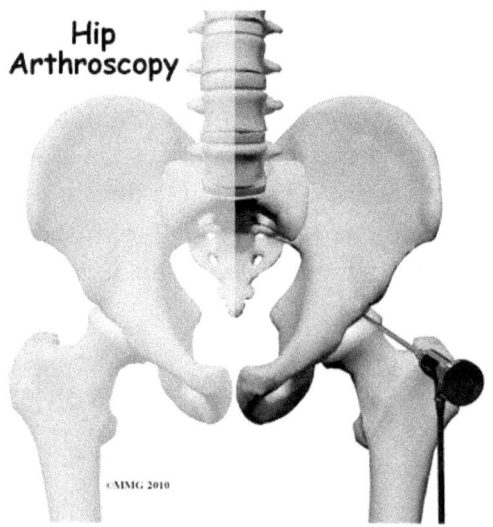

WHAT TYPES OF DISORDERS DOES HIP ARTHROSCOPY TREAT?

There are few disorders that can be treated with hip arthroscopy, a labrum tear, femoroacetabular impingement, loose pieces of cartilage or bone (loose bodies), hip infection, and inflammation of the hip lining (synovitis).

CAN HIP ARTHROSCOPY BE USED TO TREAT ARTHRITIS?

It can't be used to treat the same type of arthritis that hip replacements treat. It may be possible to treat very early forms of arthritis where only small areas of the hip have arthritis. Femoroacetabular impingement is a form of early arthritis and it can be treated with arthroscopy. Some researchers believe that FAI potentially can advance to worse hip arthritis but this has not been proven. The idea that operating on FAI can prevent hip arthritis and preserve the hip is currently not proven. For now, it is only operated on if it causes enough pain.

IS HIP ARTHROSCOPY SUCCESSFUL FOR THE OTHER PROBLEMS BESIDE ARTHRITIS, FAI, AND LABRUM TEARS?

It is good to retrieve loose bodies because is it much less invasive than an open hip operation. For infections, there is not enough information to say whether it is better than an open operation. As far as surgery for synovitis, this surgery is so rare in the hip we just can't say at this time.

COMMON QUESTIONS ABOUT SOME PRACTICAL ISSUES ABOUT SURGERY

WHAT HAPPENS ON THE FIRST APPOINTMENT?

During the first appointment, you will register for your appointment. It is important to give accurate information about your address and phone numbers as well as contact information for family members who will be involved in your care. Following this, you will spend time with your surgeon and/or assistants ho will interview and examine you. Many surgeons ask patients to see a person called a "surgical coordinator" once surgery has been decided.

WHAT ARE THE STEPS LEADING UP TO SURGERY?

1) The surgical coordinator will confirm all your information
2) You will then be sent for blood work either that day or within a few days of your first visit if your medical evaluation will be done by the hospital where you are having the surgery. If your general medical doctor is arranging this, the surgical coordinator will have you make an appointment with him/her.
3) The surgical coordinator will give you a date for surgery and review all the instructions for you to follow before the surgery.
4) You may see the medical specialist and/or the joint replacement clinical director just prior to the surgery at a separate appointment.

I ALREADY HAVE MY OWN MEDICAL DOCTOR. WHY WOULD MY SURGEON SEND ME TO A MEDICAL DOCTOR IN THEIR CENTER??

The hospital medical specialist will get valuable information from your personal medical doctor, but he/she is a specialist in preparing patients for surgery and caring for them in the few days after surgery. The hospital medical specialist does not see patients after you are discharged form the hospital so you are encouraged to continue with your personal medical physician when you go home.

WHAT SPECIFIC TESTS ARE DONE BEFORE THE SURGERY?

Here are the tests that will probably be done before your surgery

Blood Tests

CBC- this is a Complete Blood Count. This gives information about red cells, white cells, and platelets. Red cells carry oxygen. A low red cell count means you have a problem called anemia. This may need to be treated before surgery. White cells are a sign of infection. If your white cell count is high, further tests may be done to look for infection in your body. Platelets are cells that help your blood to clot and stop bleeding. If your platelets are low, then you may need more tests.

Chemistry- The information from the chemistry tests gives us an idea of your glucose (sugar) levels if you are diabetic, liver health, and a few other medical issues.

Blood Type- Patients have different types of blood. If you need a transfusion we need to know your specific type.

Other Blood Tests- In individual cases, additional blood tests may be necessary.

X-Rays

Chest X-Ray- This is to make sure your lungs are healthy
More hip x-rays. Sometimes for planning parts of your surgery, your surgeon may order more regular x-rays or may even order more advanced tests such as a CAT scan or an MRI. This will give your surgeon more information that helps in the surgery.

EKG

This is a simple test done in the office to look at the health of your heart.

Nasal Swab
>We take a cotton tip applicator and touch the inside of your nose and send it to the lab to see if you are carrying specific types of bacteria there. Some patients carry bacteria that need treatment before surgery.

ARE THERE ANY OTHER DOCTORS I WILL HAVE TO SEE BEFORE THE SURGERY?

Depending upon the results of your appointment with the hospital medical specialist or your personal physician, you may need to see one or more of the following:

>Cardiologist- a specialist for problems of the heart

>Pulmonologist- a specialist for problems of the lungs

>Hematologist- a specialist for problem of the blood cells

>Vascular Surgeon- a specialist for problems of the blood vessels and the circulation to your leg

DO I SEE THE ANESTHESIOLOGIST PRIOR TO SURGERY?

Some hospitals have you see an anesthesiologist before surgery. Others choose to see you on the day of surgery.

WHAT ARRANGEMENTS DO I NEED TO MAKE PRIOR TO THE SURGERY?

>Where you live

>>When you leave the hospital after 3-4 days your will either go to a rehabilitation hospital or to home. Even if you go to a rehabilitation hospital, after 1-3 weeks

you will then go home. Make sure you have a situation at home that is safe for recovery. This includes making sure your bed is on the same floor as the bathroom.

Who you will live with

You may need more help than you think when you get home. If you live with other people, make sure they can help with food preparation, laundry, and other basic things.

How you support yourself

How you financially support yourself during recovery is important. Make sure you do all the things you need to assure your income continues during your entire recovery. Many papers for things like "disability insurance" can be filled out prior to the surgery.

WHAT GENERAL MEDICAL INSTRUCTIONS DO I NEED TO FOLLOW STARTING THE WEEK BEFORE SURGERY?

Review all the instructions from the surgeon and medical specialists. Pay special attention to which medications to stop or continue. Report all infections or changes in your health to the hospital medical specialist and your surgeon.

WHAT GENERAL INSTRUCTIONS DO I FOLLOW THE DAY BEFORE SURGERY?

On the day before surgery, review all the medical instruction again from the your surgeon or medical doctors about which medications to stop and which to continue. You may be asked to take some of your medications on the morning of surgery with a sip of water. You will probably be instructed not to eat or drink anything after midnight the day before surgery. This means you are not to have even orange juice, coffee, and even the smallest cracker. If you forget this step, make sure you tell the doctors and nurses at the hospital when you arrive. Your surgery won't necessarily be cancelled, it may just be delayed but if you don't tell anyone you can have serious problems during the surgery.

WHAT TIME DO I GET TO THE HOSPITAL ON THE DAY OF SURGERY?

The first cases of the day get to the hospital as early as 6:30 in the morning. The surgical coordinator will tell you when to get there.

ONCE I GET TO THE HOSPITAL HOW LONG DO I WAIT UNTIL THE SURGERY?

It depends. Sometimes patients wait 4-5 hours in the hospital before the surgery. This is because surgeons can't perfectly predict the time of all the operations before yours. Occasionally they need to do other tests right before the surgery so it is very helpful for you to arrive early on the day of surgery.

AFTER THE SURGERY IS OVER, WHERE DO I GO AFTER THE OPERATING ROOM?

Patients go to the recovery room that is also called the Post-Anesthesia Unit or PACU. Some patients who are very sick may go directly to the Intensive Care Unit (ICU) or Cardiac Unit (CCU). You will stay there from 1-6 hours. You will then either go to a regular floor in the hospital or to the ICU or CCU.

WHEN CAN MY FAMILY OF FRIENDS VISIT ME?

This depends on the hospital. In some, most family friends can see you in the Recovery Room. After that the hospital has specific times of day when family and friends can visit.

WHAT CAN I EXPECT IN THE FIRST 24 HOURS AFTER SURGERY?

The first 24 hours will be a time where all the doctors and nurses will be concentrating on your general health and managing your pain. You will have a lot of tubes going in and out of your body. You job during this time is to rest and make sure you tell the doctors and nurses everything you can about how you feel.

HOW IS MY PAIN TREATED?

Doctors use many methods to treat your pain to keep you confortable. These methods can include pain medications through an intravenous, injected, or taken by mouth. It is important you speak to the doctors and nurses about how well your pain is managed.

WHAT WILL THE NEXT FEW DAYS LOOK LIKE?

You will probably get out of bed on the first day and start physical therapy. The goal is to get you safe in transferring out of bed, walking a short distance, and maybe doing some steps. A hospital discharge specialist will be speaking to you about plans for going to a rehabilitation hospital or home. Arrangements will be made for either of these and for equipment you may need. Also you will leave the hospital with information about all your appointments after discharge.

AFTER I GO TO A REHABILITATION HOME OR TO MY OWN HOME, WHEN DO I COME BACK TO SEE MY SURGEON?

Some patients come back two weeks after surgery to get stitches or staples removed. Other patients have this done either at a rehabilitation hospital or at home with a nurse that visits your home. After that you will see your surgeon at 4-6 weeks after the surgery.

HOW OFTEN DO I HAVE PHYSICAL THERAPY AFTER I GET DISCHARGED FROM THE HOSPITAL?

If you go to a rehabilitation hospital you will have physical therapy there. When you go home from the rehabilitation hospital, you will have either an appointment to go to a physical therapy office or a physical therapist will be sent to your home. If you go home from the hospital, then you will have a physical therapist sent to your home for a short time and eventually you will have appointments to go to a physical therapy office.

WHAT SPECIFIC THINGS SHOULD I WORRY ABOUT AFTER I GET HOME?

Follow all the instructions from your physical therapists about how to safely transfer from the bed or from chairs and what positions to safely keep the hip in. Review all the instructions from your surgeon and medical specialist about your medications and all your appointments. If you have any problems breathing, or experience chest pain, leg pain, leg swelling, or wound drainage, or any thing that worries you, do not hesitate to call 911 Emergency Services to come to the hospital.

WHAT IF I HAVE QUESTIONS AFTER I LEAVE THE HOSPITAL?

You will leave the hospital with contact information for many people who can help you. Keep this information handy so you can find it when you need it.

A FEW FINAL STATEMENTS FROM THE AUTHOR

Taking care of patients is a privilege and an honor. I want to thank you for the trust you have placed in me by reading this book. I welcome any and all suggestions for this book and other topics you may be interested in. If there are some questions I may have left or please pass them along to: http://www.jointsaregood.com.

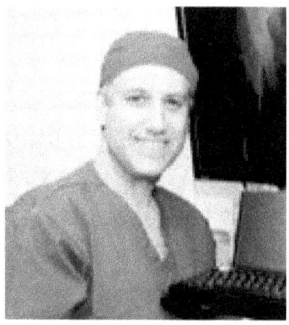

Dr. Kirschenbaum

Dr. Kirschenbaum has a unique and notable career as a surgeon, educator, computer entrepreneur, and healthcare leader. He has previously served as the Executive Director of Medscape Orthopedics and as a Community Health Editor of WebMD. He is currently the Chairman of Orthopaedic Surgery at Bronx-Lebanon Hospital Center in New York.

www.ingramcontent.com/pod-product-compliance
Lightning Source LLC
Chambersburg PA
CBHW051722170526
45167CB00002B/767